A
WOMAN
IN
RESIDENCE

A WOMAN IN RESIDENCE

Michelle Harrison, M.D.

Random House New York

Library of Congress Cataloging in Publication Data
Harrison, Michelle.
    A woman in residence.

    1. Harrison, Michelle. 2. Gynecologists—United
States—Biography. 3. Obstetricians—United States—
Biography. 4. Residents (Medicine)—United States—
Biography. 5. Women physicians—United States—
Biography. I. Title.
RG76.H37A38   618'.092'4 [B]   81–19160
ISBN 0–394–51885–3   AACR2

Manufactured in the United States of America

98765432

First Edition

To the women

who entrusted me with their care

at Doctors Hospital—whose forgiveness I ask

for the times I did as I was ordered

The setting of this book is Everytown, so named because the stories I tell are repeated in virtually every hospital throughout the country. The particular hospital in which I worked, and the doctors who taught me, were no worse than elsewhere. In fact, they may have been better. The problems I describe are not specific to any one medical community, but are endemic to the field of medicine.

ACKNOWLEDGMENTS

To the following friends and relatives who
during the living and writing of this book
provided me with encouragement, support and
criticism while adding to the fullness of my life:
Aaron, Abigail, Agnes, Alice, Ann, Annie,
Barbara, Becky, Bobbie, Bonnie, Carrie,
Charlie, Cynthia, David, Denise, Diana,
Dorothy, Eli, Elaine, Ellie, Emily, Enya, Eric,
Ethel, Eva, Eve, Francie, Gabriel, Gena, Gene,
George, Helen, Heather, Isa, Jane, Jenny, Jerry,
Jessica, Jesse, Jon, Judy, Karen, Katie, Lalitha,
Lenny, Lilian, Linda, Lise, Lonnie, Maggie,
Mary, Mary Beth, Mary Kate, Matthew, Missy,
Mitch, Nadesha, Nick, Nicola, Noni, Norma,
Pam, Pat, Peter, Phoebe, Phyllis, Rebecca,
Ruth, Sam, Sara Jane, Sarah, Shirley, Sol, Trudy,
Valery and W.C.

To Susan Griffin, whose book, *Woman and
Nature,* helped to validate for me that I spoke a
language different from the others at Doctors
Hospital.

To my editor, Charlotte Mayerson, for her
commitment to this book and to women's
health. She often helped me to articulate my
thoughts without ever trying to change them.
Working together has been productive as well
as pleasurable.

A
WOMAN
IN
RESIDENCE

I dreamed I was back at the hospital standing in a large white room. Steel shelves lining the walls held drums of a liquid which I understood was going to be given to everyone there to consume. Somehow I discovered that the drums were filled with the poison curare. I knew that we were all going to be killed. I was trying to figure out whether anyone else knew about the poison and whether there was anyone who would join me in fighting what was about to happen. Frightened but calm, I decided that I could take the poison, spit it out and pretend that I had swallowed it. Heather, my six-year-old daughter, was somewhere in the hospital. I figured out that I could also protect her by instructing her to spit out the curare surreptitiously. But there were many other children in the hospital. I had to save them, too, and I was trying to reach their mothers to warn them of the poison so they could protect their children. I kept trying to dial numbers but nothing was happening. Appearing before me and then dissolving were the faces of prominent obstetrician-gynecologists I had known. Each would come slowly toward me, enlarging, smiling menacingly, and then fade . . . to be followed by the next. I knew in the dream that they had planned it all and were going to kill us all.

I am a thirty-nine-year-old physician. I graduated from medical school in 1967. As a feminist, family physician and medical-school faculty member, I was one of many people in the late seventies who were challenging the way in which women were being treated by the health-care system. Attending home births, writing and lecturing, presenting testimony in Washington for HEW, the FDA and consumer groups, I still felt limited by my lack of specific expertise and training in obstetrics and gynecology—even though I had my board certification in family practice.

At the age of thirty-five, when my daughter was five years old, I left teaching and practice to become a resident in obstetrics and gynecology at Doctors Hospital, a prestigious teaching institution in Everytown, USA. I had sought and found a part-time position, which required my working up to seventy hours a week for half salary, or $8,000 a year. Part-time residencies had been developed to help physicians who were mothers obtain further training and still take care of their children.

In the end I was not to spend the four years in the hospital I had planned. I left because I had discovered there the poison of my dream, the poison inherent in obstetrics and gynecology as it is practiced in this country and abroad.

This book is the record of the time I was a resident. It exists because I am a diary keeper and have been since I was a young girl. In recent years, instead of writing in small thick journals, I switched to a tape recorder, both to save time and to use more creatively the time I spent driving to and from work. In Everytown, my tape recorder on the car seat beside me became at times an almost human companion, to whom I unburdened myself at the end of the day, and to whom I bid goodbye as I entered Doctors Hospital each morning.

Chapter One

I had wanted to be a doctor for as long as I could remember. I also wanted to be a mother. It seemed to me that doctoring was a form of mothering, that nurturing and healing came from the same energies, from the same center of my self that wanted to mother.

I applied to medical school knowing from advisers and other students that "I want to help people" was an unacceptable answer to the question "Why do you want to go into medicine?" I learned to say at interviews, "I find it interesting," or "I would like to combine research with practice."

In medical school I quickly found out that caring was not part of the curriculum; indeed it was discouraged. Patients, primarily black and Puerto Rican, were bodies on whom we, white and privileged, practiced. Racism among the doctors contributed to the treatment of patients as objects. My medical school memories are of patient after patient for whom I cared, but whom I felt helplessly unable to defend from the impersonal nature of hospital care.

Nancy, a seven-year-old child I admitted to the hospital one night in my final year, was one such patient. She was quite sick and was diagnosed to have a tumor of the pancreas, which is extremely rare and with which none of the doctors in our hospital were familiar. There was a surgeon at another hospital, three blocks away, who had published a paper on his experience with eight of these tumors, but because Nancy was a good "teaching case," our physicians were determined to do the surgery on their own. I had an ominous feeling about her fate, not just because of the inexperience of the surgeons, but because Nancy was being used for teaching purposes by several different departments, with the result that many unnecessary tests were being performed on her.

Two days before her scheduled surgery Nancy's parents asked me, "She's going to be all right, isn't she?"

"I don't know," I answered, trying to find ways to let them be aware of my concerns. So I told them, "What she has is very serious," wishing instead I could say, "Take her out of here and get her to people who know what they are doing!"

"The doctors seem to be good . . ." In the father's voice were both statement and question.

"Yes, but this tumor is so rare that no one in this hospital has ever seen it before. In fact, it is so rare that there have been only a few reported cases, and those were described by a doctor at City Hospital." That was as obvious as I dared be.

"Well, we have to trust the doctors. They must know best." The discussion was over.

Nancy went to surgery two days later with at least twenty people in the room. The surgery seemed to go well, but as the child was being taken from the operating room, her blood pressure fell dangerously low. At first the drop in pressure was ignored because it was assumed to be related to the removal of the tumor, but suddenly there was panic as the doctors realized Nancy's belly was swelling. The surgeons quickly reopened her abdomen, and as blood poured out, they tried to locate the knot that had loosened, the blood vessel that had not been tied securely. When Nancy's heart stopped, the surgeons slashed open her chest and tried to force her heart to pump. There was blood all over, Nancy's blood all over, and after a while they gave up and said she was dead.

I wanted to leave school that day, to leave medicine forever, to take myself as far as I could from the people around me. It wasn't only that the child had died—her illness in itself was life-threatening; it was that she died because someone wasn't careful enough. In fact, no one had been careful with her since she arrived at the hospital. I blamed myself for not having tried harder. Nancy's family invited me to the funeral and stayed in touch with me for years afterward.

Staying sane in school meant saying to myself, "I'm not like them. I do care. I am different. Someday I'll be out of here and able to do some good." But those thoughts also left me very isolated. I walked a thin line between what I believed I should be doing as a human being and what my role as a medical student required.

I was one of ten women in a class of 100 at a respected medical college, all of whom shared the same concerns about how we could combine medicine with home and family. We met to give one another support, at a time when few women were involved in feminism. In those days it was not unusual to hear women in medicine and other male-dominated fields say things like "I actually never liked being with other women," or "None of my friends are women." Hungry for role models, we tried to meet with other women in our profession, always asking the same questions: "How can one combine medicine with raising a family?"; "How did you do it?"; "Why did you not do it?"; "What were your conflicts and resolutions?"; "Are you glad or sorry?"

A pediatrician, mother of three, said, "It's easy. Anyone can do those 'animal things' the first few years. Your children don't need you until they are older and can talk."

A gynecologist advised me, "Have your children early and get it over with. That way by the time you are practicing, you don't have to bother with little children."

Other women, when asked questions like these, answered in hushed tones with an air of secrecy. Women doctors weren't supposed to talk about children. In a male world, where children were not a fit topic of conversation, I referred to these women as "closet mothers."

I worried about how I would fit it all in. I didn't think raising

7

children was doing those "animal things," or if it was, I still wanted to do them. I wanted to mother my children and I expected to use mothering in my work.

Psychiatry had become a passionate interest for me because it seemed to promise that I would find effective ways of using myself to help alleviate pain and illness. I did my internship in a community hospital on the New Jersey shore where I rotated through all the medical services, but I also spent time in a child-guidance clinic. Delivering babies at night on OB, walking along the beach with a troubled teen-ager during the day, I developed a sense of what I might achieve as a physician.

Two years of residency training, however, left me much less certain that I wanted to be a psychiatrist. Still being taught not to care, I was told by a supervisor, "Psychiatry is a science. If, in talking, the patient gets better, fine, but that is not your goal. Your goal is to understand how the mind works." No one was ever accused of "not caring."

Although I was considered talented in my work, I myself had many doubts about what I was being taught and what I was doing. Because I felt that in our close scrutiny we were missing some of the meaning of mental illness, I wanted to step outside to look at it. As foster mother to a teen-ager for a year, I had discovered that in the isolation of the mental hospital, we often failed to understand the complexities of real life, real emotions, real relationships. Humbled by the experience of living with a troubled and misbehaving adolescent, I was aghast at the advice I had so easily given to parents who had sought help with their children. I learned the obvious—that real life experience does teach us and change us.

"Maybe I'll return when I'm sixty, when I might have some answers" was what I jokingly said when I decided to leave.

My teachers were upset that I was "leaving" and expressed hope that I would return to the program. They did, however, share with me their two major criticisms of my work: I had difficulties with authority and I could not be counted upon to carry out orders with which I disagreed.

I left with the sense that I was parting from a disturbed community—and that was not only because of the patients. Staff and patients seemed to me to share in the mental illness, much as prison guards and inmates share a jail mentality.

I didn't find a place where I could practice medicine as a caring physician until I moved to South Carolina, where I was to work in a comprehensive health program that primarily served a rural black population. I opened a clinic on St. Helena, one of the coastal islands between Charleston and Savannah. There caring was acceptable, and I thought I had found a permanent place for myself.

I made house calls to comfort the dying and the families of the dying. I delivered babies and took care of them and their mothers. Sometimes I worked around the clock, but there seemed to be a purpose in what I was doing. Thirty to fifty patients came into the clinic each day, many of whom had never seen a doctor before.

When I first moved to South Carolina I looked forward to being more casual at work, perhaps to dressing in jeans and sandals. The day I opened the clinic many patients came to see me, some just to say hello and welcome me to the island. They came dressed up, though, the old ladies in hats with tiny veils and in dresses that were obviously their best. The old men came in suits. The children were immaculate. I knew I couldn't wear jeans, that it would be disrespectful. I never went without a bra in South Carolina, and I wore a dress to work each day.

Within months of our arrival in South Carolina, my brief marriage fell apart and my husband left. I found myself alone, pregnant and scared. Friends and family wanted me to return home to New Jersey, but I felt incredibly vulnerable and terrified that if I left now, I wouldn't be able to get a job because of my pregnancy. In addition, I had committed myself to my work in South Carolina, and I didn't want to abandon it. I stayed on at the clinic, working until the hours before my daughter's birth. When I was in my eighth month Heather's father had heard of my pregnancy and had called. During a long and painful phone conversation it became clear that reconciliation was not possible. We were officially divorced shortly thereafter and I've not heard from him again.

I had been trying to conceive for a year and had begun to despair of ever being pregnant. The week my husband and I separated, my menses was delayed, and when on a Friday evening it came still another time, I cried. But the next day it stopped, and the next day it started again, and continued this way for ten days.

"Doc, I've been spotting for ten days. What could it be?" I was at work and getting a corridor consultation from a colleague, the only obstetrician in town.

"Maybe you're pregnant, Michelle."

I shrugged, hiding the hope even from myself.

"Why don't you give a urine to the lab? You've nothing to lose."

The possibility that I was pregnant was thrilling but it also gave me a sense of panic because, two days before, I had admitted a baby to the hospital with a rare viral disease known to be dangerous to women in their first trimester of pregnancy. Although I asked another doctor to take care of the baby I'd admitted, I still worried throughout my pregnancy that I had infected myself and my child.

The bleeding continued on and off, and when I questioned my doctor he'd say, "Oh, don't worry, it probably means that you've already miscarried." No one was willing to believe that I wanted this pregnancy.

"But how did *you*, a *doctor*, get pregnant?" the program director asked.

"The usual way," I told him. His attitude was not as unusual as it sounds. A woman in medical school with me was once asked by a nurse, "Do women doctors have periods?"

Heather arrived in the early morning hours of December 3, 1972, propelled out of my body with a push I felt I had practiced for years. In the first moments after her birth, I knew that I wanted to be with her. I had saved enough money to hold me for a while and I would not go back to work until I wanted to or had to.

In the months ahead, sitting at the window of the small house I rented, looking out at the Beaufort River, nursing my baby from the rocking chair I'd bought years before for "when I have a baby," I felt total peace. I loved the lack of anyone else's demands. I liked knowing what to expect. Jokingly I described the difference between myself and my married friends thus: "I don't have to live with the illusion that someone is going to come home at five o'clock and make my life easier."

It was lonely, though, and at times frightening. Often Heather and I were alone for days at a time. The phone didn't ring, nor did anyone come by. My worst fantasy was that something would happen to me and it would be days before anyone would come by and find my baby. If I died, she could starve before anyone found her.

A year later the woman who was my secretary told me, "Don't get too close to that child! You'll only get hurt." It seemed that everyone was telling me that. There is something threatening to outsiders about a mother and child close to each other. Women are supposed to stay home, but they aren't supposed to be *too* tied to their babies. I was tied to Heather; I was free to be tied to her because there was no one else in my life who could lay claim to my time or attention. My life felt suspended but complete for the moment; this was the time to saturate myself with my baby, partly because I knew it wouldn't always be this way.

"Don't spend so much time with her," I was told. "You're spoiling her," I was warned. Why did anyone care so much? Why did my closeness with my baby produce such fury in others?

I said, "I want to be with her until she is bored with me and seeks others because she wants other company."

"You're making her too dependent," they warned me. "She won't be able to leave you."

I wanted Heather to be strong when she faced the world, and although I wouldn't always be able to protect her, I could start helping her learn to feel strong.

At first it was as though Heather was a person only I had

created. Then there were differences: words she didn't learn from me, ideas that came from within her. I wondered at this person who had come to be with me. She looked different, too. Her blue eyes and fine blond hair contrasted with my dark eyes and coarse black hair now streaked with gray.

"What pretty blue eyes you have, Heather," a friend said to her when she was two.

"No, I have brown eyes like my mama," she replied and burst into tears.

Since my eyes are dark, and since most of our friends were black, their eyes and those of their children were dark. Heather, wanting to be like me and like everyone else she knew, would cry whenever her blue eyes were mentioned.

"You know, you really do have beautiful blue eyes, Heather," I told her one day, "but I have an idea. Let's trade eyes."

"How can we do that?"

"Here," I said, pointing first to my eyes. "I'm giving them to you, and now I'll take yours." It was like the game of stealing noses we'd played so often, and she laughed. After that, when someone spoke of her blue eyes, she'd say, "No. I have brown eyes. I traded with my mama."

We traded dads when she was almost three.

"Who's my dad?" she asked one day when I picked her up at the day-care center shortly after we moved up North.

"Who's been asking, Heather?"

"My teacher asked me and I said I didn't know. Do I have a dad?"

"You had a dad a long time ago but he went away. Remember I told you about him once?"

She was silent. I had told her once before, about a month before while we were out on the bike, but she hadn't been ready to hear me.

"I have an idea, Heather. Remember we once traded eyes? How about if we trade dads?"

We were in New Jersey staying temporarily with my parents, and Heather was close to them both.

"You mean I could have Poppy?"

"Sure, I'm grown up now so I don't really need a dad anymore, and Poppy's a real good dad. He could be yours."

Poppy became Heather's dad, fulfilling the role of father. He even picked her up at the day-care center so she could show him off to her friends, and he still stands in at official functions requiring the presence of a dad. He calls her, writes to her, and is able to express love in a less conflicted way than he could when his own children were younger. One Father's Day Heather teased me, saying, "You don't have a dad to give a present to."

Heather had a dad and I have had the ongoing pleasure of raising her alone.

Life was different for me at home with an infant. People who had, when I was a practicing physician, valued and sought my opinion now asked me to make sandwiches for their meetings. I was asked to act as hostess to out-of-town visitors and to "drop them off" at the health center. Treated as though my brain had atrophied with the onset of motherhood, I thought, If this is how it is for me, with all that I have already done, what must it be like for other women?

Feminism clicked for me in a South Carolina grocery store one day. I was there shopping, with Heather perched on my hip, when the store manager came over and made a pass at me. I was very angry: grocery store managers don't make passes at lady doctors. When I placed an ad in the local paper to try to form a consciousness-raising group, the newspaper's owner-editor called because he thought I was trying to place an ad for some sort of orgy. When he realized what I meant he said, "Oh, you mean as in women's lib." The ad was printed in his paper with "women's lib" in parenthesis. A group of us went on meeting and came to support one another. Eventually we formed a NOW chapter and became involved in local politics.

Eventually I wanted and needed to work, to prove I could do it. So, with my baby in a backpack, I volunteered to do free school physicals in the local school system. Having convinced the people in the comprehensive health program that it was possible for me to work that way, I was rehired into the program to work, at first part-time, then full-time. I hired Mae, a woman who had raised eight children, and in a van, which served as a daytime sleeping and eating place for the baby, the three of us—Heather, Mae and I—went off to work each morning.

It was a wonderful way to be both mother and working woman. It's not that I was with my child all the time, but I was accessible to her, and she to me. If I worked late, she was with me in the van. She and Mae played, took walks, visited people down the road, gathered pecans, and made friends with patients in the clinics.

There's a story of someone asking, "Who's Dr. Harrison?," and their being told, "You'll know her by the trail of raisins." Though it looked very casual, in fact all my resources seemed to go into keeping the system working.

My memories reappear in vignettes. I was walking along a street in our small South Carolina town. Heather was in a backpack, a rare sight in those days when most babies were carried in plastic recliner seats with metal handles like shopping baskets. Walking in the streets was rare too. As we went by that day, people opened their doors and stared. I remembered my childhood and the times I had looked at someone who was eccentric, and wondered what it felt like to be like that. I thought to myself that day in South Carolina, I have become eccentric, certainly for where I live. It felt okay for me, but it didn't feel okay to raise Heather there. I didn't want her to be the child of the town eccentric.

We stayed in South Carolina until Heather was two and a half years old. I had risen in the administration of the program to become the director of Health Care Services, heading a department with 150 employees and a $2 million budget. I also continued to see some patients in the clinics. Then problems developed in the program which made it difficult for me to stay on. Tensions around both sexism and racism were mounting, and my sense of belonging was shaken. I was basically a single white woman living in a small Southern town working for a black poverty program. I had become involved in most of the community projects there, chairing the day-care-center board, raising money, serving on advisory committees, but I remained an outsider.

When I left South Carolina I wanted a quiet, inconspicuous life, where others were doing most of the work and there weren't such shortages of the energy needed to effect change. I wanted to be someplace for a while where I wasn't so needed. I moved to New Jersey primarily because it seemed important that Heather be close to her grandparents. Hoping to re-create the work and child-care arrangement I had had in South Carolina, I placed an ad in the New York *Times,* in which I advertised for a job anywhere in the New York–New Jersey area with on-site child care. The ad resulted only in a few obscene phone calls. A hospital I located which had just given up its on-site child care had decided, "There was too much demand for it." Then, giving up on finding such a situation, I enrolled Heather in a nearby day-care center. She loved it immediately, and I was able to get several part-time emergency-room jobs. Heather was proud to have a "school" to attend. At eight in the morning when I stopped at my parents' house between jobs to take Heather to the day-care center, I'd discover her clothed in a long dress, bracelets, a hat, sunglasses, a couple of scarfs, and clogs, which were a passion of hers, ready to go to school for the day.

I worked at three hospitals simultaneously, trying to accumulate the money for a down payment on a house, since I yearned now to put down roots. Our household consisted of Heather and me, and of Missie, a black-and-white long-haired terrier-type dog I'd gotten from the SPCA twelve years before, along with Toodles, a mini-schnauzer left over from my marriage, and Cari, a tiger cat whom I'd paid $10 for when I was a resident in psychiatry.

I found a large old house I could afford, and Heather and I, with our animals, moved in and invited a few friends to live with us. The house needed a lot of work just to make it habitable, but we all rebuilt, plastered and painted rooms. It turned out to be very colorful inside, for anyone willing to help out got to choose the colors used. Finding a job was no problem because I was willing to work in emergency rooms and clinics. Since I enjoyed most the part of practice that involved taking care of people, it was fine with me. As long as I wasn't trying to climb a ladder, I could find gratifying work.

"Family medicine" was a new specialty, which under its "grandfather clause" allowed physicians in practice who took the requisite continuing medical-education courses to pass an examination for board certification without having to take a family medicine residency. Determined to obtain this specialty certification, I took courses, studied and passed the examination. I began teaching at a local medical school and at a residency program where I both supervised residents and saw patients myself. Because my salary came out of teaching money, I was able to enjoy spending enough time with patients (i.e., I was not compelled to be cost-effective through the practice). The teaching scared me at first and I was unsure of myself, but I came to enjoy my work both with the students and with the patients.

Life was fairly peaceful. Heather's day-care-center hours were similar to those of my work. Often we had mornings at home together; I would take her on my bike to the center, and then I worked for the afternoon. I became more involved in the women's health movement and there found a group of women who were responsive to my feminism, my feelings about motherhood, and even my medical knowledge. Being a physician has often isolated me from the people to whom I have felt closest. For the first time, both my feminism and my work became a unified part of my life.

Years before, when I was still a resident in psychiatry, I had attended home births, but when I tried to tell my friends at work about what I was doing, I was usually warned that I could lose my license. It upset me that women were having babies in a field unattended, so I did it anyway. My first home birth, in a trailer in Maryland, was also the first time I had ever been alone with a woman throughout her labor. It took hours. There were no nurses, no shifts, no system to shield me from how long having a baby really takes. I remember opening my obstetrics book, examining the curve of labor charted on the page and feeling reassured, for the hours of the woman's labor were no longer than the hours of the curve. It only seemed longer because I wasn't used to being with the woman all that time.

When I moved to South Carolina, I didn't think about home births. There, I was taking care of a population which had just turned away from the granny midwives. Women wanted to give birth in the hospital. They wanted anesthesia, not natural childbirth. They did not breast-feed, even if that meant taking the baby home to an inadequate diet.

Our society was teaching them that almost anything was better than "old-fashioned" breast-feeding, and these mothers were committed to providing "the best" for their babies. Breast-feeding didn't regain acceptance in that community until after I had my child and was seen nursing her.

In the midst of New Jersey affluence, though, women were having babies at home without anyone in attendance, so I was again forced to confront my fears of becoming involved. After sitting on the fence for a few months, I knew that if I really believed a woman had the right to choose, I should be helping her do it safely. Little of my life remained unaffected by my decision to attend births, although there were not many actual hours involved. For example, it was necessary to give up emergency-room work, when someone's life might be endangered by my inability to be present. A woman delivering at home must have her doctor or midwife there or she is without trained help. There aren't other nurses or doctors passing in the hall who can step in and help. Always on call, I carried a beeper wherever I went. At night my sleep took on a vigilance that was a part of my work, including dreams that warned me when there was a difficult birth ahead.

Heather came with me to some of the births; her official job was to kiss the baby after it was born. Sometimes she waited in another room; at other times she was actually present for the birth. Within the growing home-birth movement, enough children have attended home births that at a national childbirth conference I once did a workshop for children who had been present either in their role as siblings or as the children of those of us who attended women at home. Children see birth differently from adults. They say, "You see, as the baby starts to come out, it turns its head and then it twists the rest of its body so there is room," and while the children talk they demonstrate to one another how the baby makes its way out. They describe the baby as an active participant both in the timing of birth and in the process of being born. "Babies like to come out when it's dark because it's more like inside the mother."

The births were a source of great pleasure for me, but also of fear. With each one that went well, I wondered how I could have been so worried. When things didn't go well, I agonized over what I should have done differently.

Although my official duties at the medical school were to teach family medicine, I also lectured on women's health care, and especially the rights of women to give birth as they choose. Appointed to the New Jersey State Medical Society Committee on Maternal and Infant Welfare, I sat with heads of OB departments throughout the state discussing such issues as midwife privileges. I accepted my function as a bridge between orthodox medicine and a community which trusted little of what medicine had to offer.

In spite of my good intentions, though, I was still suspect in the lay community because I was a physician. Originally I had planned to attend home births to support the midwives, but as it turned out, I found myself much more alone than I had anticipated. The fear surrounding home birth had affected midwives as well as physicians.

"Home birth is child abuse" was the statement coming from

the American College of Obstetrics and Gynecology (ACOG). Throughout the country, doctors attending home births were being threatened with loss of both hospital privileges and malpractice insurance. Residents attending home births either had been expelled from their training programs or were being threatened with expulsion. Legislation to limit midwife privileges was being introduced in many states. Midwives were being charged with murder if a baby died after a home birth.

Eventually, however, some competent and dedicated midwives and I began to work together and to give one another support in the face of increasing pressure to refuse our services to women. At about this time it became clear that I, especially because of the growing publicity about my work, would not be able to go on attending home births and still work within teaching institutions.

I was a family physician, not an obstetrician. If a woman I was taking care of developed any complications, I had to turn her over to others who, although more trained in the technological aspects of medical care, rarely shared my political or moral views or those of the women I treated. I wanted to do more obstetrics in the hospital as well as at home. Sometimes at the medical school, counseling students about their future, I found myself wishing I were younger and had the chance to get more training.

The development of part-time residency positions around the country began to render my hopes more attainable. Up to now I'd been stopped from going on with my training because I knew that a full-time program was more than I could manage as a single parent. Another reason I was reluctant to take more training was that I didn't believe it was possible to give the kind of care I wanted to give in a hospital. Every time I walked into a hospital, I changed, without wanting to. I became cooler, more removed, less human, more antiseptic. Patients changed too, in ways that made them turn over their destinies to professionals like me.

The birthing of a young woman named Anna gave me the sense that I *could* work in a hospital and still be myself. Anna was only eighteen when I attended her birth, and her husband seemed about the same age. When Adrienne, a nurse who worked with me, and I first arrived at the house, Kurt confessed that they hadn't practiced the childbirth exercises and he seemed frightened because he didn't know what to do. Relieved that he was not expected to "coach" his wife, he was able to be there solely as support. There is something absurd about expecting a young male, who will never experience childbirth, to be able, after six lessons, to "coach" a woman through labor and childbirth.

The young couple were living with Kurt's parents, who, along with other relatives, hovered outside the bedroom, anxiously awaiting all news. Anna labored for many hours, but then for some time she made no progress. She was a small woman with what seemed to be a large baby. A decision was made to move her to the hospital, with everyone in agreement and seemingly quite relieved.

We went to a nearby hospital where, although I did not have privileges, I did have an informal agreement that I would stay with Anna. I took her in and remained with her while she labored many more hours. The obstetrician, Anna and I agreed to postpone x-rays, since within the safety of the hospital we could just watch to see what happened. Our nurse Adrienne worked in this hospital at night on obstetrics, so she was able to assist in relations between the nursing staff and me. We didn't have privacy, because there were several nurses curious about what we were doing, but Anna didn't mind their presence.

Most important, though, was my decision not to leave the room for any reason at all. I did not take calls and there was no communication between the obstetrician and myself that did not include Anna. No conversation outside the room aligned me with the staff separate from the patient. I stayed locked in her room as if we had been at her home.

Anna was pushing and having a hard time. She tried several positions—on her knees, then standing and pushing. She stood at the side of the bed, with Kurt beside her applying pressure to her back when she wanted him to, while I stood in front of her so she could lean on me. She was leaning and breathing. We were all breathing with her. As she leaned forward, I placed my hands under her thighs to give her more support so she could bend her knees and put some of her weight on my hands. And then suddenly I realized that her feet were no longer touching the floor and that the full weight of her body was resting on my hands, in my arms. I held her that way while she pushed her baby.

The rest of the birth was as beautiful. She delivered her baby up on the bed finally, with Kurt sitting cross-legged behind her and holding her, with Adrienne listening intermittently to the unborn baby's heart beat, with me doing perineal massage to ease the passage out, with the obstetrician and the nurses watching and learning.

Reassured by this experience that I could sustain myself against institutional intimidation, I felt able to seek more training within a hospital. Strengthened by Anna's birthing, I felt I could become an obstetrician and that my hands and arms could still hold women in labor.

Chapter Two

When I started to investigate potential programs, I found that few hospitals offered part-time residency positions, and none I could find actually had a part-time resident in obstetrics and gynecology (OB-GYN). To a letter of inquiry I wrote to a hospital which must have been mistakenly listed in the part-time registry, this reply came back: "We do not offer part-time residencies ever. Please note that full time is twenty-four hours a day."

An interview at another hospital—where I didn't go—went as follows:

CHAIRMAN OF DEPT. OF OB-GYN: Why don't you send your child away to live?

ME: I can't do that.

HE: If you aren't willing to give up your child, you don't deserve to be an obstetrician-gynecologist. Dr. Harrison, your problem is that you lack motivation.

Doctors Hospital, in Everytown, was well known in the Midwest for its intent to provide humanitarian care to patients.

At an interview at Doctors Hospital:

DR. WALTER PIERCE: I'd be willing to offer you a position right now, pending receipt of your credentials.

ME: There's a hooker.

HE: What's that?
ME: I have a child.
HE: That's no hooker.
ME: And I want to do it part-time.
HE: That's a hooker.

Dr. Pierce, an accomplished GYN endocrinologist and head of the Dept. of OB-GYN at Doctors Hospital, was known for his liberal attitude toward women in training. This resulted in a higher than usual percentage of women residents in his department, but even so, he was uncertain he wanted to take anyone part-time. A full-time program at his hospital ranged from ninety to one hundred and forty hours a week. It was a schedule I didn't think I could manage as a single parent. We negotiated for a long time and Dr. Pierce finally offered me a position that was two-thirds time for half salary. I would have to work out the specific hours with the chief residents, who would be directly responsible for my daily activities.

Although I had met with Dr. Pierce to talk about the possibility of starting training the following year, eleven months hence, Pierce now said I could have the job if I could be in Everytown to start work in four weeks. He had just fired a resident that week, so he needed someone at once. With no certainty that the offer would be good the following year, I felt I had to take advantage of this opportunity.

I left Pierce's office astounded because I had the offer I had wanted, in a city where I had friends, in a program with a chairperson who was supportive of women, in a residency program with other women. And because I was going to one of the finest and most humanitarian of hospitals, the difficulties would at least be fewer than elsewhere. All I needed to do was gather letters and credentials from all the places I'd been, negotiate with the chief residents about the schedule, and move halfway across the country. Each piece seemed manageable.

There would be three chief residents—all women—each for a period of four months during the year. They had started together three years before, and now, in their final year of residency, they would take turns being chief residents. Carol, a woman I knew from work in the women's health movement, was currently the chief. She had almost four months to go.

Carol was the person who had urged me to call Dr. Pierce to talk about a position, telling me, "He likes strong women."

"He offered me the job!" I reported to her ecstatically later in the day.

"I know. I've already talked with him. We have to talk about the hours."

When she found that the other residents were opposed to my coming into the program part-time, Carol had had to do her own negotiating about me. I knew I would need the support of at least the chief residents if I were to succeed at all. Jackie, who would be chief in the spring, wanted to talk with me before any final agreements were made since, as she told me that evening, "I have to live with the decisions that are made now. I'll be your chief in the spring."

Jackie and I talked on the phone. She was worried and doubtful the arrangement would work. "You know, politically I'm in favor of what you are trying to do, but I don't want to be left to do your work." However, she was surprised that the schedule tentatively worked out by Carol and me called for me to work many more hours than she had expected. "My husband once knew a part-time resident in opthalmology who was never there and never did her work," she said.

Jackie went on, thinking out loud as she tried to create a schedule that would best help the hospital but would not be full-time. Interspersed with her listing possible duties, shifts, days of greater surgery, were her doubts about my plans. "I don't think you can really do this if you have kids," she said. "I decided a long time ago that I'd have an abortion if I got pregnant while in training.

"A lot of the others will resent you," she added.

"I know that."

"They can make it tough for you."

"I know that, too; that's why I wanted to be sure that at least you and Carol felt all right about my coming here. I don't expect it to be easy."

"Everyone here is overworked, so there will always be excess demands on your time. You're going to have to be able to protect yourself. No one will ever be satisfied with what you do because there is always more work to be done."

Jackie finally presented a plan. I would come in five mornings at six o'clock and see patients until eight. On Monday and Tuesday I would then be free to leave for the day. If I was to be on call for the night, I would return to the hospital at five and stay either until morning or through the next day. On Wednesday, Thursday and Friday I would work from six in the morning until six o'clock at night. I would take night and weekend call every sixth night, as Carol and I had already agreed.

"But can you take orders?" Jackie asked as though needing to satisfy one more doubt of hers; Dr. Pierce had already asked me the same question.

"Jackie, I know the rules of the game. I think I can take it. I've told myself I'll take whatever I have to in order to make it through. I'm giving up a lot to be here."

We were both worn out by the end of the phone call. Jackie had to be at work at six, and soon I would be there too. The following morning I was on the phone sending telegrams to schools, training programs and jobs where I had been, authorizing them to send letters to Dr. Pierce.

Fran and Laurie are the friends I was visiting in Everytown when I met with Dr. Pierce. Both are women's health activists I knew from conferences around the country. I had first met them in New Jersey when they spoke there, and then I turned to them for support as pressure mounted for me to stop attending home births. Although I didn't know them well, we shared a sense that we would be close friends if we ever lived in the same city. We had planned this visit so we could finish some of the conversations that were forever being interrupted by plane schedules, conference schedules and work.

Fran's response the previous May when I first told her what I wanted to do had been, "But you can't do that! They'll destroy you. You'll either come out thinking like they do or you won't make it through." We were in a car going to dinner from a board meeting of the National Women's Health Network in Philadelphia. Fran was navigating while I drove. With only four blocks to go and others waiting for us at the restaurant we got lost, circling numerous streets neither of us knew while Fran tried to talk me out of what I wanted to do. She didn't think I could survive, and she didn't want me to do that to myself. Failing to dissuade me, she added, "Well, if you're going to do it, Everytown is the place for you to be. At least you have support there."

Laurie, a slight young woman in her mid-twenties with a singular passion to improve the health care of women, was excited at the prospect of having someone whom she trusted trained in obstetrics and gynecology. The night I was offered the position we celebrated at Laurie's house. My mood was dampened somewhat by a call from New Jersey that Missie, my dog of fifteen years, had died that morning. Her death, though not unexpected, was tremendously painful. She had been a constant companion for most of my adult life.

By the first of August, Dr. Pierce had received my records, and he had notified me that he expected me in Everytown in three weeks. I was still obligated to work another two weeks in New Jersey, which gave me one week between jobs. School would be starting for Heather in the first week of September, by which time I needed a place to live, a school and after-school care. Critical to the entire plan was that I sell the New Jersey house, since I was counting on that profit to support me at least through part of the residency.

I made a list:

sell house	finish job
buy house	notify patients
child care	move

Heather was to have entered kindergarten in New Jersey, but was old enough for first grade in the Everytown area. I was uncertain about which grade to place her in and was unable to get help in that decision because it was August. Some of the local schools had after-school programs, but because it was summer and these programs were all parent-run, no one could give me information about them. I was told that some of the after-school groups had long waiting lists, but no one knew at which schools. Finding a house depended on the after-school care available.

When I first planned to do this training, I had expected to have six months to a year in which to make the move. Ideally I would have found a living situation with other adults and children so there would be a sharing of child care and so Heather would not be so alone while I was working. But when it all happened so fast, there wasn't time to find or create such a household that could be expected to be stable. Living with others is difficult, and those arrangements always take enormous amounts of emotional energy and time if they are to be successful. Finding a place to live was again complicated by our having a dog. Toodles, the mini-schnauzer, had gone to a friend, but we still had Maggie, a sheltie who shadowed Heather and was an integral part of our family, and Corny, a brown, black and white guinea pig. Rental ads all read: "No pets."

I finally found an independent after-school program that picked up children at four schools and kept them until six-thirty. I told the real estate people that I needed a house in one of those four school districts. The major asset of the house I found was that Heather could walk out of the kitchen door and be in the school yard. If all went well we could be in the house by Labor Day. A mortgage was approved after I demonstrated that the anticipated profit from the New Jersey house would support me during the residency.

While I traveled back and forth to the Midwest looking for a place to live, arranging child care, etc., friends began preparing the New Jersey house for sale and for the move. The bright sky-blue ceilings and green banisters enthusiastically painted in the early days of making the house livable were now being covered over with plain white.

Heather would stay with her grandparents for the two weeks before we closed on the house. Once we moved in, Fran and Laurie would take turns getting Heather off to school in the morning until I found someone to live with us. When I had to work all night, Heather would stay at Laurie's house.

I worried about what this would be like for Heather. She didn't want to move. She didn't want to leave her grandparents, her aunt, her baby cousin, her friends. She didn't want to leave Susan, a woman who had been living in the house in exchange for some child care, and who I had hoped might move with us. I worried about the disruption, and about what the next years would be like for her. This was the time that I had anticipated, that I had told her about when she was a baby, that time when I could no longer be with her so much. I hoped she felt loved enough and that her sense of herself was strong enough, that she would be all right.

Doctors Hospital is a university-affiliated teaching hospital with both private and "service" patients. The private patients have their own physicians, referred to as "attendings," with residents having varying degrees of control over their care. The service patients, those who in years past would have been referred to as "ward" or "charity" patients, come through the clinic or emergency room and do not have their own doctors. Most of these are black or Hispanic. The residents have control of their care. Both private and service patients are studied in the teaching program.

Residents assigned to gynecology take care of emergencies and perform time-consuming examinations and procedures for the attendings. In return for performing those tasks, the attendings allow the residents to learn surgery on their patients. This is possible because the teaching of surgical skills occurs when the patient is under anesthesia—and thus unaware of who is doing the surgery.

Residents on obstetrics follow women in labor, see both private and service patients on daily rounds, and take care of prenatal and postpartum patients who have complications. In return, the residents are allowed to do deliveries, sew episiotomies, and to assist or even perform Caesarean sections, tubal ligations, and other procedures on these patients.

Doctors Hospital also employs midwives to take care of pregnant and birthing women. Midwife literally means "with woman." The last years have seen a resurgence of midwives attending childbirth, which had become the province of physicians in this century. Certified nurse midwives are registered nurses who are also graduates of midwifery training programs and are certified by the American College of Nurse Midwives. Lay midwives, however, have come to their work through a variety of paths, usually including a period of apprenticeship with another practicing midwife. Many lay midwives become skilled at attending the large numbers of women who are choosing not to go into the hospital but, rather, to give birth at home —with or without anyone there to help them. In most states, lay midwives are practicing illegally but meeting the demand of a population alienated from the medical system.

Although certified nurse midwives have been trained to manage labor and delivery on their own—and are doing so in many areas of this country and others—at Doctors Hospital they are directly supervised by attending physicians. Other than that there was a delivery atmosphere modified by their presence as supportive women, it was often difficult to distinguish a midwife-attended birth from any other.

The relationship between residents and midwives was not clearly defined. The residents took part in the labor management of the midwives' patients, but then usually stepped out at the time of delivery. Ultimate responsibility for the patient, however, rested with the attending physician.

Within the residency program there was a complex hierarchy. All residents are MDs who have already served a year of internship either in this or another hospital, and are now taking this four-year training to become specialists in OB-GYN. There are junior residents, senior residents and chief residents, and on each level there are varying degrees of autonomy, authority and deference given or demanded. At each level there is also fear of the person above: the chief resident is responsible for what all the others do, and subject to the anger or praise of Dr. Pierce, a tall muscular man with thick black hair and penetrating eyes.

Dr. Pierce's department is accredited for sixteen residents, four at each level, but there are rarely sixteen at any time, since residents are prone to transferring, breaking down and being fired. Fewer residents means more work for each resident, but it also means less competition for surgical cases and deliveries.

I was accepted into the program at the second-year level, having been given credit for my board certification in Family Practice.

THE GYN SERVICE—GOING TO THE OPERATING ROOM

I, as a second-year resident, was to be on gynecology for the next ten weeks. Carol was chief resident, Richard in the third year, and Barbara the first-year resident. Together, the four of us took care of all the gynecological patients in the hospital.

Richard, tall, fair, a loner, was quiet and reserved, rarely speaking unless directly addressed. Barbara was slightly more friendly. Having only begun the residency in the past month, she was already unhappy and thinking about quitting. She felt lonely and out of place in this Midwestern city, and complained that she wasn't getting enough surgical experience. Barbara had beautiful long dark hair, which was never out of place, even after a night on call. She was furthest from the stereotype of a woman doctor, and on most days could have been chosen for a beauty pageant.

We met each morning on the GYN floor at six o'clock. From six to seven-thirty we made "work rounds": before we saw the patients we reviewed vital-signs sheets, on which were recorded the temperature, pulse, breathing rate and blood pressure of each patient on the unit. We checked each woman's intake and output sheet to see how much fluid had been consumed and excreted, and then we went to see each one.

On the first morning I followed Carol, who was warm and friendly, managing to give each woman the sense that there was all the time in the world in which to answer her questions. She hid the urgency she felt about time until she was outside the room and out of the woman's hearing. Often Carol, short and slender, her thick blond hair in a single braid, white jacket over slacks and blouse, looked and sounded incredibly young and girlish. Sometimes, though, there were dark lines and a look of deep worry on her face.

Most patients were either preoperative or postoperative. We changed dressings, took out sutures or the metal staples that were sometimes used instead of sewn stitches. We listened to lungs. We put stethoscopes to bellies, listening for the intestinal rumblings that heralded the return of proper functioning after surgery. We asked patients whether they had passed gas or moved their bowels, which helped us to decide when to stop intravenous feedings and begin liquid or solid foods. If there had been a fever in the past twenty-four hours, we began searching for the source of infection, culturing urine, sputum, skin, wounds, throat, cervix . . .

We immersed ourselves in information about each patient and returned to the nurses' station to make notes on charts and write orders for tests we wanted. Orders had to be on the chart by seven every morning, or the lab technicians wouldn't draw the blood samples, and one of us would have to do it. We had to know who each patient's attending physician was and how that attending wanted his or her patients to be managed. Did the attending allow resumption of feeding with the return of bowel sounds or the passing of flatus? Did we need to consult with the attending before we made such decisions? What role did we play in the care of that doctor's patients?

The day's plan for the patient had to be established and all the work done during those rounds because we would be tied up in the operating room (OR) for most of the day.

Seven-thirty found us in the cafeteria, giving patient reports to the chief resident over breakfast. An extra muffin or doughnut became a reward for a bad night or an anticipated difficult case in the OR. We had thirty minutes in which to review all our patients and to show what we knew or didn't know. Carol began with the report from the person who had been on duty the previous night. New admissions were described to the rest of us, and then we discussed the complications of the night. Hurriedly we went through the card file of the approximately forty patients and discussed each woman's condition, progress, lack of progress, and plans.

By eight o'clock we were in the operating room. Once in the OR, how did I feel? I felt important. This was not the first OR I'd been in, but this one carried all the atmosphere of the major university of which it was a part. There is something about a uniform, too, that makes one feel important. My whole being reeked of my station. I was an insider. I looked just like the others. I had a place, a job, and I was being taught the secrets of medicine. If we had expressed our feelings of elitism, we might have said, "How terrible never to see the inside of the OR, never to have a role in the drama there." I was ashamed of the power I felt in that room, ashamed of what I was becoming, and yet I was also enjoying it.

The operating suite covered two floors. Upstairs were the changing and locker rooms, separate for men and women. There were two lounges, a smoking lounge with a coffee urn and microwave oven, and a nonsmoking room with more chairs and dictating machines and a telephone to the outside. Beyond the lounges and dressing rooms was a central hall with stairs leading down to the actual operating rooms. A large stainless-steel rack in the hallway held masks, hats and booties.

Carol took me to the women's changing room, where there

were two large racks of clothing stacked by style, color and approximate size. Blues—for men and women—were for surgery, either in dress style or as pants and top. Grays were for taking temporary trips out of the OR without having to put on regular clothes. Carol and I changed into blues, shedding white coats, clothes, watches, rings, and went outside to the stainless-steel rack. Booties came in two sizes: too big and too small. They fit over our shoes and helped keep the floor of the operating room from being contaminated. The booties had little black straps hanging out the back which were supposed to be tucked in against our skin to ground us and prevent electrostatic explosion in the presence of inflammable anesthetics, but no one ever tucked them in. They either trailed behind us or were ripped off. I assumed our operating room had special flooring that made the straps unnecessary. The hats came in various shapes to cover our hair. Some for men with short hair were merely tallish skull caps. Others looked like a loose, full kind of shower cap. For men with beards there were hoods that covered both their heads and chins. The masks were put on as we headed down the stairs to the OR, and they had to be in place by the time we went through the OR door. Once inside the OR we could not be paged and all messages had to come through the OR secretary. I was suddenly conscious of being cut off from the rest of the world, and especially from my child. I had to hope that she was all right and that if she wasn't, someone would persevere in getting a message to me.

The staircase down to the OR seemed magical. It was common practice, and one in which I joined, to grab the handrails and jump the last three or four steps into the OR area.

Through the door at the bottom of the stairs was a large central nurses' area with desks, supplies, phones. Twelve individual operating rooms opened into this area. On one wall hung a huge glossy white laminated board on which each case was listed by room number. A cardboard box beside the board held magnetic name plates. We'd go first to the board, find our case, and then slap our magnetic name plates onto the board where they hung suspended, defying gravity.

I was in the OR with my name now hung on the board, officially announcing that I belonged. Everyone in the operating area was fully clothed in blues, hat, booties and mask. It was unsettling to meet people there for the first time. It took me months to put together the slits of eyes and skin with whole faces and bodies.

After Carol and I found the room where our case would be, we went to the sinks to scrub. The sinks were large shiny basins with foot pedals to control the water spouts and disinfectant dispensers. Over the sinks were instruction sheets on the various methods of scrubbing. The sheets looked old and showed the effects of years of soap and water splashed on them.

Scrubbing is a ritual that begins with a short rinse with plain water: hands are wet first, and then the arms, which are always held so that the water goes down toward the elbows, not toward the hands. Then a new, disposable brush, presoaked with pHiso-Hex or iodine, is taken from a dispenser at the side of the sink. The cover is ripped off, while taking care not to drop the brush, which becomes slippery from the wet hands. The scrubbing begins in a pattern from fingers to hands, then arms, always with the water running down toward the bent elbows, so that hands are always held up toward the ceiling, toward God.

To get from the sinks into the rooms meant going through a door, using one's rear to open the door and one's leg to close it. The task was to stay clean, to go into the OR without touching anything, without helping anyone. It was hardest not to help, not to reach as an instrument was falling, not to pick up a towel left on the floor. Hands must stay as they are, reaching upward, arms bent at the elbow, water dripping to the floor.

Next the gowning begins. The nurse tosses you a sterile towel for one hand, and then a second towel for the other hand, each one being dropped to the floor as it is used. Then the gown is put on carefully so that no part of the outside touches one's body or anything else. Finally the gloves are put on, with scrubbed hands making a dramatic dive into the gloves being held open by a nurse. To touch anything is to "break scrub"—which means you have to repeat the entire procedure.

Only the territory above the waist is considered sterile, so one's hands always have to be held above the waist. The most common position is with arms crossed over the gown, sterile gloves to sterile gown, as in a bilateral pledge of allegiance. There we stood, covered by hats, masks, gowns, gloves, booties, with arms crossed, waiting to begin.

Every precaution was taken to keep the room and ourselves as sterile as possible, but sick surgeons don't stay home. (As doctors we are not allowed to be sick. We just cough and sneeze through our sterile masks.)

THE D&C

A D&C is the "bread and butter" of gynecologic surgery. That's how it was described to me over the sinks one day as the attending surgeon and I were scrubbing to do the operation. The procedure is a dilation (D) of the cervix, and then a curettage (C) or scraping of the uterus.

The D&C patient is usually a middle-aged woman with irregular vaginal bleeding, for which she gets her womb scraped out both for diagnosis and for cure. Many women simply stop having this bleeding problem after a D&C, but no one is sure why. It reminds me of exorcism. It may be that the ritualistic and mysterious aspects of the procedure add to the success of the exorcism.

Whatever my theories, I was there at my first D&C to learn how to do the procedure. I paid careful attention to the details of how I would be expected to conduct myself within the few weeks it would take for me to master this operation.

The patient awaited surgery in the "holding area," a large room with space for four stretchers against each of the walls, and curtains which could be drawn between each stretcher for some minimal privacy, if necessary. It was here that patients usually had their intravenous fluids (IVs) started, and where they waited to be called into the operating rooms, having given up their clothes, eyeglasses, jewelry and teeth before they left their rooms upstairs.

Patients left the holding area on their stretchers and were wheeled along a wide corridor that surrounded all the operating rooms and that opened into each room separately. At the door of the room where she would have her surgery, the woman was transferred to the operating table, which had been brought out into the hall. As part of the effort to keep the room as clean as possible, the stretcher from the holding area was not allowed into the room. I wondered for a moment what it must be like for the woman on her table, being wheeled into this alien atmosphere: a large room with chrome-encircled spotlights suspended from the ceiling on long arms; racks of supplies along the walls; hanging bottles on IV poles with long tubing as yet unconnected; tanks of gas with colored round dials and indicator needles; monitors with blank flat lines traveling across their screens, waiting to be given signals to measure and count. The woman, naked under the sheets, often cold in a room heated for the comfort of those of us dressed in many layers, hears of herself in the third person. She catches bits and pieces of our language which may or may not be important or related to her.

"Do you have my favorite dilators ready?" a surgeon asks a nurse.

"No, they're still in the autoclave being sterilized. Do you want us to hold up the procedure until they're out?"

"No, I'll use what you have," he tells her.

The woman on the table worries. Why are some his favorite? Are the others as good? Will he operate as well with the substitutes? Her fate in the hands of us in the room, she tries to sort out the importance of the random remarks she hears.

The summer I was nine years old I broke my arm at camp swinging off the cabin rafters. Not wanting to get into trouble for my activities, I stoically told no one about my fall until late at night when the pain was enough for me to ask for aspirin. I was then rushed to a hospital, where my arm was set and I was admitted for the night. The nurse who put me in a bed showed me a buzzer clipped to the pillow and said, "Push this little button if you need anything." Then she added, "Don't worry, we won't pump out your stomach if you call." She was referring to another child in the ER who had been screaming as his stomach was pumped, but all I could remember were the words "pump out your stomach," so I avoided touching the buzzer. I couldn't be sure if it would or wouldn't happen to me. It must be that way for a patient on an operating table.

"Bad"—a word the woman on the table catches in a conversation. Was a nurse saying her case was bad, or wasn't bad? All that remains is the word without the context. The sounds of the operating room are a fusion of medical terminology, commands, deference, interspersed with words of everyday life. The patient is an anonymous body on a table, a living cadaver about to be put to sleep.

The same summer I broke my arm, I saw a rabbit "put to sleep." For years I was terrified of being "put to sleep." I wasn't sure where death took over and when reawakening was no longer possible.

Nurses place electrodes on the patient's chest so her heart can be monitored. A grounding plate, covered with green gel, is placed under the woman's back. Almost invariably, she winces because it is cold.

Carol and I come into the room while all this is happening. Carol takes the patient's hand and tells her she will be fine, and as she introduces me, I wonder what this woman will ever remember of what she can see between my mask and hat.

The anesthesiologist, seated at the head of the table, is in charge of the preoperative procedures around the patient. Carol and I are told, "You may scrub now," and we leave the room. The patient is given a drug through her IV that puts her to sleep and then one that paralyzes her muscles, including those of respiration. A tube is put in her trachea so that a machine can breathe for her. The monitor counts the rhythmic contractions of her heart.

The anesthesiologist signals that the woman's legs may now be put up in stirrups. The nurses make sure the woman is correctly on the table, not too far toward the head or foot. Two nurses, in unison, one on each side, lift the woman's now heavy legs so that her feet can be put in the stirrups which are at the bottom of the table, about twenty-four inches apart. Once in this position, because the woman is paralyzed, her legs fall out to the side.

As Carol and I watch from the sinks, she instructs me on what we will be doing. I keep thinking about anatomy class when I was in medical school. When we got to the pelvis on our cadaver we made a joke of the body and hung the legs from the ceiling. We made a joke of death and a joke of private parts. In the OR we hang legs on stirrups. We put the woman to sleep so she is loose and we hang her. A woman with her legs in the air cannot fight. She cannot protest the remarks about her fatness, her hair, her scars, the shape of her labia, the size of her clitoris. She cannot pull her legs together to protect herself. I stop my thoughts in order to learn what I have to know and to go along with what I have to do.

Carol and I watch the nurses scrub the patient first. A disposable tray with sterile sponges and bottles of disinfectant is opened. The nurse takes the first sponge, and starting at the labia, wipes the brown staining liquid out along the thighs. Once a sponge is used on the outer portion of the body it cannot be returned to the center of the operative site. Before the sponge is thrown away, it is used to scrub the anus. The nurse's scrub ends with her patting the entire area dry with a sterile towel.

Carol now takes the smaller tray with three more sterile sponges on sticks and soaked with disinfectant. Her first sponge goes into the vagina, and remains there with the yellow plastic stick protruding out. The second sponge is used on the labia and then wiped outward about five inches along the thigh. The first sponge is then taken out of the vagina and passed down along the anus. The third sponge is used to repeat the scrub of the inside of the vagina.

Draping begins: the first drape, a large gray-green sheet, goes under the woman's buttocks, the second and third along the thighs, not quite meeting at the labia. The last sheet is on top of the woman, meets the two leg sheets at the pubis, and completes a ring of sterile sheets around the vaginal opening. There is now a complete sterile field consisting of her drapes and our gloves and gowns.

The anesthesiologist had signaled when we could begin the second scrub, and now we await the signal to begin the operation. Although the woman is asleep, if she is not at a deep enough level, she will straighten her legs and fight us when we put an instrument in her vagina.

We empty a patient's bladder as a routine, using a thin catheter which is passed through her urethra, since a full bladder could interfere with the vaginal exam.

The exam under anesthesia (EUA) is performed because we can more easily examine the pelvic organs, since the woman's abdominal muscles now offer us no resistance. The patient is examined by Carol, by me, and by a medical student who is watching us. We note the results of the exam on the chart. The anesthesiologist tells us we may begin the procedure.

The D&C is simple but it still scares me, since there is always the possibility of harming a woman. A speculum, an instrument used to stretch open the vaginal walls, with a heavy-weighted handle is placed in the vagina, thus pulling the lower portion (floor) of the vagina downward without anyone having to hold it. Carol takes a long flat L-shaped instrument that looks like a bent ruler and places it in the vagina, her left hand pulling upward with it and stretching the vagina open so that the woman's round cervix can easily be seen. A tenaculum, a thin instrument about sixteen inches long, with tiny teeth on the end, is used to grasp the upper lip of the cervix, allowing us to place traction—a pulling force—on both the cervix and uterus. Carol has me hold the tenaculum so I can feel how much traction is exerted. Then she removes the L-shaped instrument, leaving the weighted speculum in place.

The os, or opening of the cervix, is dilated by using a series of increasingly wide metal probes. Carol shows me the different ones on the instrument table, put out so surgeons can use their favorites. Some dilators are more or less traumatic to the cervix, some are easier to use, safer, look more elegant. She shows me which are her favorites and I know I will start with those when I am on my own.

We insert into the uterus a sound, a thin flexible metal rod about fourteen inches long, to see how deep it is and at what angle to insert the dilators. Then we take the smallest of the tapered dilators and begin to stretch the os. Carol puts in a dilator while I take it out and hand her the next larger size. As I remove each dilator I can feel how the uterus slopes. We dilate until we think the os is open enough to admit the curette, a long thin instrument with a curved cup at the end with tiny teeth as on the edge of a saw. If the os is not yet wide enough to admit the curette, we dilate it more. The curette is then passed through the os into the body of the uterus, and its sharp edge is used to scrape the lining as it is withdrawn. Then it is inserted again at a slightly different angle and is withdrawn again. The bits of tissue are deposited on a piece of gauze that is resting on the weighted speculum. The fragments of uterine lining will all go into a specimen bottle to be examined in the lab within the next few days.

Tissue is taken from all corners and then randomly from the cavity of the uterus, the curette making a to-and-fro motion. The scraping continues until there is a gritty feeling to the entire lining of the uterus. It is the gritty feeling which is sought and which Carol makes sure I feel. It is called the "cry of the uterus."

This time it is we who signal the anesthesiologist that we are almost finished so the level of anesthesia can slowly be decreased. We take the fragments of tissue from the gauze and place them in a bottle with preservative. Then we remove the tenaculum and examine the cervix to be sure it is not bleeding excessively either from our curetting or from the teeth of the tenaculum, which sometimes pierce a vessel in the cervix or tear the os. As the weighted speculum is removed from the vagina, the woman's labia come together. We signal that we have finished by sweeping the drapes up off the patient and depositing them either in a large bin or on the floor, leaving the rest of the cleanup for the nurses.

One of us must stay with the patient until she is in the recovery room, but now time is spent filling out pathology forms for the specimen; writing operative notes, recovery-room orders, and notes to ourselves about what care this woman may need later. The nurses will call us to help transfer the patient to a stretcher to go to the recovery room, but our attention is no longer with this woman. We are getting ready for the next case.

LAPAROSCOPY

On the third day I learned laparoscopy. "Lap" is for loins, loosely including the abdomen; "scope" is an instrument for viewing. Thus, laparoscopy is the use of an instrument for viewing the inside of the abdominal cavity including the uterus, Fallopian tubes and ovaries. During laparoscopy the tubes can be "tied" for sterilization, either by burning them with an electrode or by putting rings on them which block sperm from traveling through them. Laparoscopy is often referred to as bellybutton surgery because the laparoscope is put through a hole made in the perimeter of the navel. It is also called Band-Aid surgery because usually only a Band-Aid is needed to put on the incision. This makes the surgery seem insignificant.

Laparoscopy is simple surgery if you know what you are doing, if nothing goes wrong, if the equipment is working, if the nurses know how to run the equipment, and if the patient's insides look and behave as they are supposed to. I was assisting a private attending Dr. Owen, on my first laparoscopy, keenly aware of the loss of Carol as my teacher. Dr. Owen's large frame and pedantic manner contrasted with Carol's slight build and gentle manner of teaching.

Much of surgical procedure is repetitive. The patient is brought to the OR, given anesthesia, scrubbed and draped. The nurse does the initial scrub of the abdomen and perineum, and then the surgeon takes over, repeating what has just been done, but also scrubbing out the vagina. Two sets of drapes are put over the woman, thus establishing the vaginal and abdominal operative sites.

After the woman's bladder is emptied with a catheter, she is examined under anesthesia. If she is to have a D&C as well as laparoscopy, the D&C is done first. Dr. Owen did the D&C, explaining to me, "I do it to be sure the patient isn't already pregnant, since we are going to tie the tubes." He added, "I like to do whatever I can while I'm in there, anyway. You never know what you might find."

The D&C finished, Dr. Owen leaves the tenaculum attached to the cervix and then attaches it to a canula, a long thin nippled instrument, which is placed into the os. The handles of the two instruments are now hooked together, and with a sterile towel draped over them are used to manipulate the uterus during the laparoscopy. The weighted speculum at the base of the vagina is removed, allowing a 360-degree rotation of the instruments, which are now protruding out of the woman's vagina.

"In gynecologic surgery, the vagina is defined as dirty," Dr. Owen tells me as he takes off the pair of gloves he is wearing over his first pair. I, too, take off my gloves; I did not do the D&C, but I examined the woman under anesthesia and thus contaminated my gloves. Some surgeons also change their gown after touching the vagina.

We move to the woman's abdomen, I on her right, he on her left side, allowing him greater use of his right hand in manipulating the laparoscope. Taking a small pointed knife from the nurse, Dr. Owen makes a stab wound into the outer ring of the woman's bellybutton and hands the knife back. He takes a long thin needle, and as he grasps the patient's abdominal skin with his left hand, he instructs me, "Lift up now as hard as you can," and I can hear the strain of his lifting in his voice. Struggling to keep the woman's skin from sliding out from my gloved fingers, I grasp it more tightly and pull upward. While we both pull, he pushes the needle through two layers of abdominal tissue and into the abdominal cavity. He tests his success by putting a drop of water on the open end of the needle and watches to see if the water disappears as he opens the needle valve. "We're in!" he tells me triumphantly.

I maintain some traction on the woman's abdominal skin while he hooks up the needle to a machine which will pump carbon dioxide into the woman's belly.

We relax and watch the gauges on the machine. "I like to put about three liters into the abdomen before I go further," he tells me, noting that the machine already read one liter when we turned it on. The woman's abdomen begins to inflate.

Periodically Dr. Owen reaches over her abdomen to tap it and hear how it sounds, then motions for me to do the same. Her abdomen begins to sound hollow as I tap and then I move my fingers to her upper abdomen where her liver is, and where for years I have percussed the sound of liver dullness marking out the boundaries of that organ. The usual dullness now becomes tympanitic as the carbon dioxide separates her liver from the abdominal wall, against which it usually lies. When the gauge reads four liters and there is hollowness throughout her abdomen, Dr. Owen swiftly removes the needle, sealing the woman's abdomen closed in its inflated state.

"Trochar," he calls, and the nurse hands him a spikelike instrument, about eight inches long, with a pyramidal-shaped end. Surrounding the shaft of the trochar is a fiberglass sleeve with a piston valve at its end. Now that the woman's belly is taut, it is much harder to grasp her skin. As we both try, I feel that I am trying to pull her into my chest. The table is too high for me, so I don't have good leverage for what I am trying to do. "Harder," he tells me, and I try harder while he begins pushing the spiked end of the trochar through the incision we made previously at the navel. Then, with a twisting motion that seems to include his arm and his shoulder for strength, he forces the instrument through her abdominal wall. Suddenly there is no resistance and he relaxes. "Listen," he says, and as he releases the piston valve, I hear the sound of escaping air. He closes the valve, sure that we are in.

"Hose," he calls, and I hand him the hose, which he attaches to the valve of the sleeve. Then he turns to watch the machine. The nurse turns the dial to "Automatic," so the machine will slowly pump air into the abdomen to replace what leaks out during the procedure. As the trochar is removed from the sleeve, there is a momentary *whish* of air before the valve closes.

Dr. Owen now guides the shaft of the laparoscope through the sleeve of the trochar into the woman's abdominal cavity. The laparoscope is a tube about eighteen inches long and about a centimeter in diameter. It contains a magnifying lens and a connection for a light source. Its function is similar to that of a periscope, except in this case we are looking in from outside instead of looking up from under water.

"Lights out," he says to the nurse. "Tilt, please," he requests of the anesthesiologist. The room becomes darkened except for the light coming from the windows to the next room. The anesthesiologist begins turning the crank at the head of the table and the woman's body is slowly tilted backward so her head points toward the floor and her buttocks toward the ceiling, making her intestines fall downward against her diaphragm instead of into her pelvis. Because of the woman's position, the surgeon looking into the pelvis from the bellybutton is actually looking upward. The room is dark, the woman is tilted, and only Dr. Owen can see what is there.

"It looks fine in here. I have good visualization of the uterus. I can see one tube but I can't see the ovaries clearly." He reaches with his left hand through the woman's legs to the instruments protruding from her vagina and pushes them downward toward her abdomen as though trying to make both sets of instruments meet inside her. He mumbles that now he can see the left ovary, and then, with a scooping motion, he moves the instruments down and as far to the left as he can, saying, "Ah, there's the other one."

"You may look now," he tells me. I lean over the table to the laparoscope, and being careful not to touch the lens and not to contaminate any of the sterile field with my mask, I take my first look in. I see wonderful red and orange and yellow, all without form. He asks if I see the uterus, tubes, ovaries, which he tells me are all right there. "Well, I see something," I tell him, wishing Carol were there with me. Dr. Owen takes the shaft of the scope, and looking through the lens, says, "You were angled too high." He readjusts the scope, looks through and tells me to look now, but in the passing of the instrument from his hand to mine, the angle is again changed. I catch a glimpse of something.

"Knife!" and a knife is in his hand. He angles the scope upward against the abdominal wall, so in this darkened room we can all see the light shining from inside the woman's belly, as he searches for an area where there is no large blood vessel so he can make a second incision. Finding a clear spot of light along the woman's pubic hairline, he quickly stabs at the place where the light shines through. She bleeds slightly.

"Grab the skin the way you did before," he instructs me. As we lift he forces a second trochar through the woman's abdomen at the site of the stab wound until there is no resistance, and he says again, "We're in." He removes the trochar, instructing me to hold my finger over the sleeve to prevent air from escaping, since this sleeve has no valve.

"Is the ring loaded?" he asks of the nurse, referring to the ring applicator that will be used to tie the woman's tubes. He goes on to tell me he prefers the rings to using cautery, which burns the tubes. "These rings are cleaner, and it's easier to reverse the procedure if she changes her mind in the future. It's almost impossible to reopen the tubes after they've been burned." I look at the ring, white plastic, about a quarter inch in size, which has been loaded into a long ring applicator with retractable teeth. As he inserts the ring applicator through the second sleeve I realize there are now three sets of instruments protruding from this tilted woman's body. There are the toweled instruments attached to her uterus and coming out of her vagina, there is the laparoscope coming out of the incision at the navel, and now the ring applicator coming out of the second incision near the pubic hairline.

Looking through the scope while he manipulates the toweled vaginal instruments, Dr. Owen brings the right tube into full vision. While I hold those instruments in place, he takes the ring applicator and explains what he is doing. "I'm grasping the tube and pulling it up into the applicator with the teeth at the end. Then slowly I release the ring and it slides onto the knuckle of the tube which has been drawn up into the applicator." His face becomes knotted and intense as he draws up the tube, then suddenly eased as he tells me, "I'm releasing the teeth so the tube with the ring on it drops back into the pelvis." He offers to show me. I look in and see a piece of white plastic attached to some tissue, and although the structures are still not clear, I am glad I've seen the ring. The procedure is repeated on the other side, so there is now a white ring on each tube.

The anesthesiologist asks if we are done but Dr. Owen says no, it will still be a few more minutes, and then invites me to come around to his side of the table to look inside. Taking the scope is now easier because I can use my right eye and my right hand. As I move the scope around, this time I am relieved that the colors have form and that I can begin to distinguish what I am seeing.

"You can wake her," he tells the anesthesiologist; although it will still take some time to finish, it will also take time for the woman to come out of the anesthesia. All of us wince at the sudden brightness when the nurse turns on the lights. For a few minutes it seemed as though the only world there was existed in the belly of the woman on the table.

The ring applicator is removed from the woman's abdomen, causing her belly to quickly deflate. At Dr. Owen's instruction, I remove its sleeve, which is sticky at first but with some pulling comes out, allowing the skin to close over the incision. Dr. Owen removes the laparoscope, and then, pressing on the woman's abdomen, forces out more of the air through the incision, removing the second sleeve as he continues to exert pressure on the abdomen. With the sleeves out, there are only two small wounds in the woman's belly with a few drops of clotted blood around each one.

"Staples!" he calls, and the nurse hands him a tweezer loaded with a staple which he uses to staple shut the umbilical incision. He calls for a second staple for the same incision, and then a third for the smaller incision along the pubic hairline. I am instructed to put on the Band-Aids.

Dr. Owen moves to the space between the woman's legs to remove the vaginal instruments. He detaches the canula from the tenaculum, then removes the tenaculum from the cervix. Using a speculum, he examines the cervix and vagina for any bleeding either from the D&C or the tenaculum teeth. "Done," he declares, sweeping the drapes off the woman's legs and dropping them to the floor for the nurses to pick up.

The patient is awakening. The tube is removed from her throat and she is placed on her side so that if she vomits, she won't draw the contents of her stomach into her lungs. She shivers, moans. With slurred speech thick with mucus from her throat and vomitus from her stomach, she wants to know if it is over and asks, "Am I okay?"

I am at the Formica shelf along the wall filling out the forms for her chart, but the anesthesiologist and nurses at her side answer her as they prepare her for the recovery room.

In a typical morning I would do three D&C's and a laparoscopy, or one D&C and a hysterectomy or other major operation.

THE WORK-UP

Afternoons were for work-ups—a term that includes taking a medical history and performing a physical exam (H&P), then recording them on the patient's chart, as well as writing orders for lab tests, diagnostic procedures and medications on the chart. Although we often needed to contact the private attending about any special orders or problems, it was the performance of the History and Physical that took the most time.

After leaving the OR I would stop at the bulletin board, where there would be tiny folded pieces of paper with our names on the outside, and the names of patients to be worked up on the inside, usually the ones on whom we would be operating the following day.

None of us could leave at night until all the H&Ps were done, so we had to manage whatever there was in the time available. All of us usually did a good job on the first H&P of the day, but by the second, third or fourth we were often exhausted and just wanted to go home.

The H&P seems like "busy work," since it has already been done in the private doctor's office. But it must be recorded on the chart to fulfill both legal and accreditation requirements. Since it is quite likely that no one will ever read the H&P or pay attention to what it says, it doesn't have to be thorough or legible. It just has to be there.

At two in the afternoon, when I have already put in an eight-hour day, I must gather my energy and interest to find out all about someone's life and health. Going to the room of my first patient, I tap lightly on the open door.

The woman, alert and healthy-looking, still in street clothes, is sitting on the bed, and she says into the phone as she hangs up, "The doctor is here." A second bed in the room is occupied by a woman recovering from surgery two days before, so I draw the curtain between the beds, a pretense at privacy.

Since this is my first work-up for the afternoon, I sit down, but as I get busier and more pressed for time and worried about getting out, I stand during the H&P. Sometimes when I had been awake for thirty-six hours I would hold the 5×8 card I used for taking notes in front of my eyes, and I could actually shut my eyes for brief moments while I listened to the patient. I could also take momentary naps when listening to a patient's heart. Closing my eyes, I could sink into the rhythm of the heart or of breathing, and napping between beats, would actually feel refreshed.

But this day I feel fresh when I go to see this patient, and she seems eager to see me arrive—a step closer to her surgery in the morning. She asks, "Will you be there for the surgery?"

"The schedule calls for me to be there, but it could still change," I tell her and then sit back in the chair to begin taking her history.

"What brings you to the hospital?" I ask. Of course, I already know exactly why she is here and what surgery is planned, but I must be able to write it in the chart *in her own words*.

Her chart will read: "The patient is admitted with a chief complaint of 'I have fibroids and the doctor says they have to come out.' " Continuing with my questions, I obtain the History of Present Illness. "When did the fibroids begin giving you trouble?" She says she has had two years of intermittent irregular bleeding and a D&C which took care of the problem for about a year, but now she has the bleeding again and it worries her. I ask more about the nature of the bleeding: Is it heavy, is there pain? What are her fears?

Gathering information for the chart, I move on to the rest of the OB-GYN history. Menstruation: When did it begin, how often does it occur, how long does it last? This information will appear on the chart in a formula as "Menarche [age at onset] × length of cycle × duration of menses," or "Menarche: 12 × 29 × 5." An added note will indicate whether she has cramps or any irregularities. I wonder at the relevance of these questions: by tomorrow afternoon she will not have a uterus and will have no more menses. The date of her last period, noted on the chart, will indeed be her last.

I ask about urinary problems, incontinence, infections, VD, vaginitis, birth control, sexual problems, then obstetrical questions: Has she been pregnant? How many times? Abortions? Miscarriages? Premature births? Nature of deliveries? Does she have breast pain? Lumps? I ask the most intimate questions of this woman, although I may never see her again.

Once in psychiatric training a supervisor wanted to know if I'd obtained some very personal information from a patient. "No, I didn't ask that question. I didn't think it was any of my business." We say that patients should always tell us everything, but that trust should be earned, not assumed. Charts are not really private, nor are we always discreet.

Written on the chart next will be the Review of Systems, so I ask about her general state of health, energy, weight, mood. I ask about her nervous system, tics, tremors, convulsions, dizziness, headaches. I go on to vision, eye problems, ear problems, hearing. I ask if she has had any problems with her chest. Frequent colds? Cough? Sputum? Heavy breathing? Painful breathing? If she answers yes to any problems, I ask more specific questions. I cover heart and blood vessels, then chest pain, leg cramps, leg swelling, fainting. Since this is a surgical service, we are careful to ask about bleeding disorders, whether the patient has any known bleeding problems and also whether she bleeds a lot when cut or when having a tooth extraction, for instance.

As I list possible digestive problems, which few of us are totally without, I try to sort out the serious from the inconsequential, especially from a surgical perspective. "Do you have problems with swallowing, vomiting, appetite, heartburn, constipation, diarrhea, hemorrhoids, food intolerances—especially fatty food, abdominal pains, nausea, etc?"

I finish with extremities and then skin. "Do you ever have pain in your joints? Have you ever broken a bone? Do you have rashes?"

"Well, I used to. Does that count?" she asks, to which I respond, "Well, no, not for this part of the history, but yes, tell me anyway," as I mark on the 5 × 8 card "Skin problem," with an arrow pointing to Past History, which comes next.

The Past History is a listing of about twenty diseases specifically asked about, including chronic illnesses, hospitalizations, surgery, and then allergies, especially to drugs and penicillin.

The Family History is the list of diseases that have occurred among her relatives. "Are your parents alive, healthy? What problems did they have, if deceased, how? Do you have siblings? What is their health?" When I ask about cancer, heart disease, diabetes, I know I have caused the woman to worry about whether she will have them because she assumes I wouldn't be asking those questions if they weren't relevant.

"Do you smoke? Drink? How much?" I ask as part of the Social History, and then for a woman, instead of "Do you work?" I ask, "Are you employed outside the home?"

The history taking completed, my 5 × 8 card is now filled with words, cryptic abbreviations, numbers and sentences, either listed or connected by arrows. Although I have asked and she has told me "everything," there is always more remembered during the examination.

This is a routine physical exam, which aside from the internal pelvic exam is done in the patient's room, since the GYN unit has only one exam room and each of us tries to use it as little as possible.

Generally the exam is done starting at the head and working downward, covering head, eyes, ears, nose, throat, all of which will be abbreviated on the chart as "HEENT—negative." I feel the woman's neck for masses and thyroid size, then listen to her heart and lungs. I feel for masses in her breasts. Resting my hands on her abdomen, I feel for tenderness and masses. Tapping, I percuss out the size of her liver by listening for the area of liver dullness. I look briefly at the woman's legs, noting veins, looking for swellings and deformities.

We go to the exam room for the rest of the exam. There, because I am a woman, I am alone with the patient. Male physicians are accompanied by nurses when they examine women internally to protect them from accusations of sexual assault; of course, that also means they have an extra set of hands to help them in the room to get what may suddenly be needed for the exam.

The exam room is small, about ten square feet with a curtain which slides halfway across, giving some privacy from the window in the door. Cabinets, counters and sink line one wall; standing in the middle is the GYN table, short, padded, with stirrups on the end.

I direct the woman to get up on the table, where she sits while

I gather my instruments. Now in a white gown and robe, she looks like a patient. Her tentative questions of me are in sharp contrast with her confident voice on the phone when I entered her room.

"Do you do breast self-exam?" I remember to ask her.

"I know I should. I just don't like to" is her response, a common one. Some women say they find it too frightening, partly because of the difficulty in distinguishing between dangerous lumps and normal breast tissue, which can at times be lumpy.

With the woman now lying on the table, her feet in stirrups, her legs covered with a drape, the light adjusted, I examine her labia, clitoris and urethra for abnormalities. Then with a speculum I examine her vagina and cervix, looking for any areas of redness, scarring, infection, abnormal glands or secretions. Following the speculum exam I palpate the woman's pelvic organs by inserting two fingers of my right hand into her vagina; at the same time, I place my left hand on her lower abdomen and try to feel her uterus and ovaries between the finger of my hands. This woman's uterus is enlarged from the fibroids, so it is easily felt. I cannot feel her ovaries, but that is not unusual when they are normal. I finish with the rectal exam, taking a bit of stool from my gloved finger and checking it for any occult blood, which could indicate intestinal bleeding.

"You can get up now," I tell the woman, offering to help her but realizing there is no graceful way to get up from that position.

She asks what I think, and I tell her, "You seem to be in quite good health, other than your enlarged uterus. I'm sure you're worried, but fibroid tumors are benign, as you know." I speak to her unsaid fear of cancer.

As we walk back to her room I explain what will happen to her for the rest of the day and evening. An anesthesiologist will see her and take some of the same history, examine her heart and lungs, and assign a risk category for her in terms of the anesthesia. If either I or the anesthesiologist discover any problems, consultants will be called.

Every patient must be "cleared" for surgery. She must have

her chart in order, lab tests done and reported, her chest x-ray done and read by the radiologist. If she is over forty, she must have had an electrocardiogram (EKG) read and cleared by the cardiologist. The resident on duty for the night will "pre-op" the patient—that is, make sure everything is done, consent forms signed, and that any consultants called have now cleared the woman for surgery in the morning. The chart must also contain an "informed consent" note written by the attending, stating that all risks of the surgery have been explained to the patient.

Leaving the woman back in her room, I return to the nurses' station, where I find a quiet corner in which to write the history, physical, summary of pertinent findings, and then recommended treatment—usually the operation, which has already been scheduled.

The order sheet is the official communication between the doctors and nursing personnel. I write "Admit to GYN," although she has already been admitted, since it can't be official until I order it. I assign a diet (she won't be fed until I order a diet), and then list lab tests, chest x-ray and EKG, all of which have already been done. I write an order, "Anesthesia to see patient," although in many instances they may be with her already or may have seen her before me. Sometimes it seems that we are doing endless perfunctory and superfluous tasks to produce a chart—which will stand up well in court.

I've promised the patient I would order sleep medication for her, so I do that. I've called her attending, who wants her to have an enema, so I order it. I order that her pubic hair and abdomen be shaved for her hysterectomy in the morning.

The chart is not written in peace. There are endless calls on my pager, questions from patients and nurses, minor or major emergencies. I write on, though, and as I write I am separating myself from this patient. It is as though I am discharging her onto paper. It is urgent that I finish and go on, because she was only my first work-up this afternoon.

Chapter Three

Monday 5:30 A.M., on my way to work   *Day 1*

Last night was the annual dinner at Dr. Pierce's house and I met
many of the residents in the program. They seem to be depressed, talking mostly about work and suicide. I left with a
good feeling about being older than they and I hoped, past
many of the turmoils of growing up.

I'm staying at Laurie's for the next two weeks, while Heather
is back in New Jersey with my parents. There is a bid on the
New Jersey house and I've gotten the mortgage on the house
here, so we should be able to move in ten days.

This morning feels like a new beginning, one I have worked
hard to create. I feel brave and adventurous but also scared.

Later

After a day of taking care of patients, scrubbing on a hysterectomy that Carol and Dr. MacDougal were doing, and then
doing work-ups, I am heading back to Laurie's for dinner and
then back to the hospital, where Carol is going to give me some
extra lessons on tying sutures. I feel so incredibly fortunate to
be getting this training.

There has been a resident rebellion over my coming to the
program as a part-time resident. Dr. Pierce met with the residents and said they had no choice but to have me here. They

were somewhat appeased when he told them I was working two-thirds time for half salary and only partial credit.

Wednesday   Day 3

"Are you married?" Dr. Owen's questions were becoming increasingly personal as we were scrubbing at the sinks before a case.

"No," I answered, after a short hesitation, trying to indicate that I wasn't going to offer any more information than I had to.

"I hope you don't mind these questions."

"No, not at all," I answered. I knew my ability to succeed here was going to depend on how I got along with attendings as well as the other residents.

"My nephew is going out with a woman medical student and frankly I'm quite worried."

"Good choice," I said jokingly, keeping the rest of my thoughts to myself.

We went through the doors of the OR, he leading, both of us with our upward-reaching hands and bent elbows, and he asked, "What is your first name?"

"Michelle."

Nurses were handing us towels to dry our hands and listening to our exchange.

"Do you mind if I call you by your first name?"

"That's fine," I told him and after a moment I asked, "What would you like me to call you?"

There was silence; he looked uncomfortable and then responded, "In this setting I am used to being called Dr. Owen."

I went about putting on my gown, and as the nurse tied the back I said, "I'll be pleased to call you whatever makes you more comfortable."

Thursday, on the way to work   Day 4

I talked on the phone with Heather last night. I miss her and look forward to this weekend when I'll be back in New Jersey.

I'm working full-time at the hospital right now, trying to build up a little equity so I can get some hours off to start Heather in school.

On the way home

My first work-up this afternoon was on a woman who is having laparoscopy for a lost IUD. An IUD or intra-uterine device, is a plastic or metal birth control device which is inserted through the cervical os into the uterus. This woman's IUD is outside her uterus, somewhere in the right side of her pelvis. It has been located there both by x-ray and ultrasound, a technique which uses sound waves instead of x-rays to form a picture. The IUD apparently perforated through the uterus after it was put in. I asked the woman what she was planning to use for birth control after this.

"Oh, I'll have another IUD put in," she said, as though surprised by my question. Noticing my surprise, she added, "I'd just like to see what another one does."

While I was with her I could hear the woman in the next bed talking on the phone about the surgery she'd had. She is an infertility patient who, during surgery last week, "accidentally" lost an ovary. On the phone she was telling someone that "the bad ovary was removed, but the good one was left in."

Both these women had such trust in the medical system.

Friday   Day 5

At first we couldn't find the IUD. When the surgeon couldn't see it with the laparoscope, he tried to find it inside the womb. While exploring the woman's uterus he accidentally perforated it with the probe. I was looking through the laparoscope when I suddenly saw a metal probe coming through the wall. When we then did a laparotomy (opened her abdominally) we could see the two holes in her uterus, one where the IUD had presumably perforated, and a new one made while the inside of the uterine cavity was explored. We finally found the IUD in the tissue around the ovary and tube, removed it and repaired the damage.

One of the surgeons realized he knew the bank officer who had handled my mortgage, and we chatted about real estate and school systems while we hunted for the missing IUD.

I had time today to go to the laundry to try on a white coat and pants. I'll be issued four sets, which are to last my stay here. Up until now I've been wearing my street clothes under a short white jacket I found hanging in the closet of the on-call room. We all wear white coats, but some of the residents wear white skirts or pants. Residents who have been here long enough to have gained or lost weight tend to have given up on their uniforms and just wear the coats. The jackets are most necessary because of the numerous pockets in which to keep papers, pens, medical instruments, wallet, notebooks, miniature textbooks and sometimes snacks.

Before leaving this evening, I took care of an eighty-two-year-old woman about to be discharged. She has a prolapsed uterus, which is falling down so badly that sometimes it protrudes through her vagina. Someone had prescribed a pessary, a rubber device to hold it up, but the pessary was too large and when I tried to insert it into the woman's vagina she screamed. I stopped, and told her I'd order a smaller one.

"My uterus has been that way for twenty years," she told me. "I don't want anything done to it. I can push it up myself."

She was in the hospital for a medical condition when the prolapse was discovered. I'm not sure she'll come back next week for the smaller pessary. Though there are medical reasons to use a pessary, many older women prefer not to have a device in the vagina.

Tuesday evening   *Day 9*

I have been on duty for thirty-six hours. Most of the night was spent working in the emergency room seeing women with gynecologic emergencies as well as nonemergencies. The work was familiar and similar to what I've done for years in family practice and emergency-room work. Richard, my chief for the night, made it difficult for me to figure out what decisions I may or may not make on my own. Each time I called to ask about a patient, I'd also ask if I was supposed to be calling him or whether I should take care of the patient myself.

"I don't mind your calling" was his perpetual answer, although it didn't address my question. Having assured Dr. Pierce I would "take orders" even from those younger or, in some cases, less experienced, I do not want to step outside the bounds of what I am supposed to do on my own.

Today I scrubbed on two D&Cs, one on a very obese woman about whom there was much joking. Anesthetized women look so vulnerable.

Sunday afternoon as I stood on the porch of my New Jersey house I realized I might not see it again. We had rented a U-Haul truck and will move next weekend. I have spent a weekend packing and there is still more to go; my friend Missy will do it for me. I have too much stuff and no time to sort out what to take or get rid of. I've loved that house, which has been a place of parties, meetings and poetry readings. It's been a resting place and refuge for me and my friends. My friends have been wonderful, though we are all sad to part from each other.

Thursday   *Day 11*

Today I scrubbed with Richard on a mini-lap, a modified abdominal tubal ligation. We began by trying to do it by laparoscopy, but when we looked inside, we saw a hydrosalpinx, a large fluid-filled sac swelling the woman's Fallopian tube. We went in abdominally, removed the hydrosalpinx and tied the tubes.

Sunday morning, on the way to work   *Day 14*

Friday afternoon we moved to Everytown. Five minutes after we began unloading the truck two girls, about eight and ten, rode by on their bikes and invited Heather to join them. Though she is only five, she learned to ride last week—just in time—and she proudly went off with them. An hour later she returned, asking if she could go swimming with them; I said that was fine if one of them could lend her a suit, since I couldn't locate anything of ours. Heather has moved in.

Friday night my friends Missy and Sandra arrived from New Jersey to help unpack and put the house together. Then last night we went to a party at the home of Catherine, a woman physician I've also met at many conferences. I finally met other members of the Midwestern Women's Health Alliance, including Diane, a woman at whose apartment Heather and I stayed when we were visiting in July. It was an evening of music, talk and food, and although I was tired, I was glad to be there.

Snuggles, a multicolored kitten, is the latest addition to our household. She joins Maggie, the sheltie, and Corny, our guinea pig. Barbara had gotten the kitten when she moved to be a resident, but she cried all the time because Barbara was never home.

Beginning this morning I will be on duty for twenty-four hours; Missy will stay at the house with Heather. I feel very taken care of by my friends.

Monday morning, on the way home   *Day 15*

Yesterday morning I arrived at the hospital to find that the woman whose hysterectomy I watched last week was going back to the operating room for the third time. Last week they took her back to remove a blood clot from the site of surgery, and yesterday they opened her and cleaned out all the clotted blood and pus, which should probably have been removed the first time they took her back.

The afternoon was spent doing work on the unit and taking emergency-room calls. Jackie, who is covering for Carol as chief resident for the weekend, came in for a while. She is a short, slim, intense woman who rarely looks relaxed. Trying to catch her attention, I said "Hello." She turned to me and said, "I have a lot of scut work for you to do, Michelle." "Scut" is work of no educational value, like drawing bloods or taking EKGs, work usually done by a nurse or technician but also done by residents in teaching hospitals. Jackie was letting me know that she had the authority to assign scut work to me. The work wasn't bad because I had plenty of time, but I didn't like being treated that way, especially by a woman with whom I expected to be friends. Her casual dress, jeans and loafers, make her authoritarian demeanor more of a surprise.

A woman who had laparoscopy last week has been running a fever for the last two days, but no one has found the source of the infection. Yesterday Barbara wanted to put a probe into the incision to see if pus drained. "The woman is infected in the incision," Barbara insisted. "It's because of her obesity." Richard claimed the infection was intra-abdominal and wanted to take her back to the operating room and open her up.

"Don't you have anything else that would explain the fever, like a cold or something?" I asked the patient last evening, partly in jest, partly because I was so frustrated at not being able to find the source of infection.

"Well, as a matter of fact, I've had a sore throat for days but no one seems intersted."

Examining her, I discovered she had a large tender and swollen neck mass. She told me she has had infections of her parotid (saliva-producing) gland before. I'm sure that is what she has now.

Richard ridiculed me at rounds this morning when I told the others what I had found, but we're still getting an Ear, Nose and Throat consult on the woman.

Late last night a woman came into the emergency room with a lot of abdominal pain and looking very sick. Richard and I argued about whether or not to admit her because he didn't think her problem was so serious, but at three in the morning he finally agreed to admit her. The two most probable diagnoses were pelvic infection or an ectopic pregnancy, which is a pregnancy in the Fallopian tube and which is potentially fatal. Richard said they would no doubt take her to surgery in the morning, and told me to go to sleep. The nurses and I were upset about leaving the woman for that long because by then we strongly suspected it was an ectopic pregnancy that had ruptured. One nurse said she thought the woman's belly was becoming more swollen; this would happen if she was bleeding internally. Instead of going to sleep, I ordered another hematocrit, a blood test I expected to show blood loss.

An hour later I woke Richard with the results. He called Jackie, who called the attending, and we rushed the woman into the operating room. When we opened the woman's abdomen, the blood came pouring out. It continued to spill out until the bleeding tubal pregnancy was located and tied off.

As I kept trying to sponge up blood—my job as the junior member of the team—Richard would tell me to stop, that I was in his way. Then a male nurse would do exactly what I had been doing, and there would be no comment from Richard. At one point, when the field was filled with blood and it seemed impossible to see anything, I reached in with a sponge and Richard slapped my hand. The nurse went on sponging. I can't let myself respond. I've promised myself I will put up with anything.

The patient did well through surgery and is expected to have a normal recovery. Jackie congratulated Richard for his good work, and especially for having quickly gotten the hematocrit which showed the woman was bleeding.

Richard will be my chief when I am on obstetrics in another month. This worries me a lot.

Tuesday   *Day 16*

This morning at breakfast rounds, Jackie seemed to be trying to pit Barbara and me against each other, referring to my having higher rank as a second-year resident, and changing her mind several times about who would do which surgery. As we were dressing for surgery, Barbara and I agreed that we wouldn't let Jackie set us up against each other. We could go along with Jackie today because we knew that the issues would disappear when Carol returns. Carol can make the same assignments or ask that the same work be done but without polarizing issues or people. In the same way that she gives patients the sense that she cares, she makes taking orders seem right and even pleasurable.

This afternoon on my way home I stopped at the school to register Heather. The kindergarten–1st grade combination (K-1) seemed the most logical place to put her since that would give everyone a chance to see where she really belongs. The principal, however, said the K-1 was full and he wanted her in the 1-2 class. I'm worried about that because, although she is five years old and of first-grade age, she hasn't been in kindergarten yet. It's so hard as a mother to know when to insist and when to leave it up to the experts.

"I'm not going to after-school!" Heather said adamantly.

"But why? You've always loved day care and you've always loved being in child care wherever we've gone."

"I'm not going, Mama. I'm not going," and this time she was weeping.

I didn't understand. She had loved the after-school center when we went to see it and to meet the teacher. After a few minutes at the center, Heather was able to tell me why she was so upset. "The kids said when I was in first grade I would have so much homework I couldn't do anything else in the afternoon. They also said that if you didn't do your homework, the teacher would hit you over the head with a book and I'm scared because I don't want to get hit."

Heather accepted my reassurance and is now looking forward to being at the center. I suspect that after a while she will prefer to be home in the afternoon with her friends, but I have a sense of relief that the center is there if I need it.

Wednesday morning   *Day 17*

There are beautiful pinks and blues and touches of yellow coming across the sky as I drive in to work at sunrise.

Finding a live-in baby-sitter will be my next project. Some days I think I can manage Heather, the house and work, but most of the time I feel pulled in so many different directions. The hours I'm working make it more difficult than most situations, but my problem is not unlike that of any working woman —especially if she is a single parent. There's never a breather.

On the way home

The woman who had the ectopic pregnancy met me on rounds this morning with, "You know, I was awake for the surgery and I can remember it." She is eighteen years old and this morning, hair in curlers, mildly distracted by the TV cartoons, she looked like a testy teen-ager.

"What do you remember?" I asked, aware that what she was saying was possible, especially with a drug which paralyzes people even if they are not fully asleep.

"I remember thinking I was at a party, and everyone was standing over me passing joints from one person to another. Then I remember being opened up, and having my blood spilling out all over and everyone looking frightened. That's all I remember," she said, looking triumphant, daring me to disagree.

"I guess you were there, but I don't remember any joints," I told her jokingly.

The joints must have been the instruments being passed from hand to hand. Her memory of the fear we felt when the blood spilled out of her was accurate.

Later in the day I mentioned her story to the anesthesiologist, who became angry and said she was crazy.

Dr. Neisel is a very old surgeon who still operates at the hospital, but with an unofficial rule that he must have a chief resident with him. This morning I scrubbed with Jackie and him, while Dr. Pierce came by to watch for a while. Dr. Neisel seemed to suspect that he was being watched closely, so before surgery, while we were all scrubbing, Jackie and I pretended that Dr. Pierce has been making surprise visits to look over everyone's shoulders.

Dr. Neisel became aphasic during the hysterectomy—that is,

he couldn't find the words for what he wanted, for the instruments he needed. He kept saying "Kelly," which is a kind of clamp used in surgery. But when the nurse handed him the Kelly clamp, he pushed it away and repeated "Kelly." At one point the nurse had handed him every instrument on the tray but he rejected each one and then reaching onto the tray himself, took a scalpel.

Trying to lighten the situation, Jackie said to him, "I just think you've got the sweets for Kelly," referring to a nurse in the OR. Jackie also kept trying to do surgery for him, since his hands weren't very steady. She'd kid him, telling him that he wasn't giving her enough teaching experience because he was doing it himself. Several times I caught Dr. Pierce's eyes and he seemed upset about what was going on.

Thursday   *Day 18*

This morning as I walked Heather out the back door and over the small hill to her school, I was overwhelmed and tearful at the sense I had of the repetition and continuity of generations. Heather was dressed up in a new skirt and a blouse her grandparents had sent from New Jersey. She was still wearing her clogs. At first she was scared in the classroom, but she relaxed and let go of me after meeting her teacher and another child. The day-care-center bus will pick her up at school, and then I will pick her up at six. I feel bad about her going right from school to the after-school program today without my being there. I'll be concerned about her all day, hoping she is all right.

This morning at five-thirty, before taking Heather to school, I went into the hospital, made rounds, and left for home again at seven-thirty. By ten I was back in the operating room, scrubbed on a laparoscopic tubal ligation.

I remember one day last year at the day-care center when a new teacher didn't show up for the first day after vacation. Since my time at the medical school was flexible, I was able to stay, but I remember other mothers who were rushing to work and couldn't stay because a boss was due back, or a class was waiting, or they simply had to be on time. Motherhood in our society means always being on the edge between two existences which rarely allow for any overlap.

Friday   *Day 19*

Usually when a woman has fibroid tumors that are giving her discomfort or bleeding, she has her entire uterus removed. Today, however, I scrubbed on a myomectomy, or a removal of the tumors from the uterus, on a woman who wants to become pregnant. The tumors look like round red balls imbedded in the walls of the uterus and bleed profusely when they are removed. The woman had two large ones, each the size of a lemon, and then some tiny "seedlings," which were also removed. The outer capsule of the tumor is shelled off, like peeling an orange, and then the bulk of the tumor is tied off in sections. It is a more difficult procedure than a hysterectomy, and seems to have a higher complication rate.

I have been practicing tying knots on napkins and furniture at home, but it is different from tying knots in surgery, where my gloves are wet and slippery with blood, I can't see well, there's never enough room in the operative site, and I'm trying to hurry.

Tuesday   *Day 23*

Laurie will pick up Heather at the after-school program and keep her for the night because I'm on duty for the next thirty-six hours. This morning when I left, I realized that no one will be home, so I left a note asking Laurie to let Maggie out once tonight and again in the morning when she drops Heather off at school. The dog is one more responsibility.

Arlene, a college student, is the only person who showed up for an interview for the job, although I had many calls over the weekend. She says she likes children and is used to them; she is the second oldest of nine. She would be able to attend her classes and still be home in time for Heather. I have to call her last reference today, but I feel almost certain I will hire her.

Dr. Neisel has been telling his patient on whom we operated last week that Jackie is the one who is taking care of her. Whenever the woman mentions my name as the one who sees her on rounds, changes her dressings, etc., he looks at her blankly. Today she called me into her room to ask when I would start my own practice, because she wanted me to be her doctor. "Dr. Neisel is getting old," she told me, as though apologetic for noticing. "One of these days I know I will need another doctor."

I have been watching a lot of D&Cs and noticing the motion used to scrape out the inside of the uterus. The curette is jabbed in and out of the vagina repeatedly, held in the surgeon's hand as if the force of the thrust is coming from his/her body. Watching the procedure, I found it difficult not to think of the word "fucking." I don't know why that style is necessary or why they aren't more gentle.

Wednesday   *Day 24*

When I am on call for so many hours, my body becomes bloated and feels out of shape. My legs are swollen and my clothes are uncomfortable against my skin.

I've hired Arlene, although I wasn't able to reach her last reference, but I need some relief. She should be at the house when I get home.

Fran called about a friend of hers and Laurie's who has just come to Everytown and needs a place to stay for a while. I offered her the spare room, so she should also be at the house when I get home.

I slept last night at the hospital between three and six in the morning, so I don't feel as terrible as I might.

Arlene has moved in and Heather is delighted to have a new baby-sitter, especially since she has been complaining about having to go to the after-school program instead of being able to come home and play with her friends. Heather is thrilled to have someone else in the house who enjoys hair fixing and dressing up. I am relieved that the constant arranging of child care is over.

Gail, Fran and Laurie's friend, was also at the house when I got home last night. She is resettling here after having been in England for the past ten years, and she may stay on at the house for a while. Fran and Laurie came and we cooked a big dinner for everyone. Home is beginning to feel the way it did in New Jersey.

On the way home

I had a busy morning in the OR with two D&Cs, a laparoscopy and a mini-lap. Dr. Catan, the surgeon with whom I was scrubbed for most of the cases, is an older, roundish, kindly man who was quite nice to me. Afterward, though, he took me aside and said, "Dear, you hold your instruments like a plumber." His criticism struck me with peculiar accuracy. Between cases I had been on the phone trying to reach a plumber about a shower leak, and had said apologetically to one, "Ordinarily I would do the work myself, but I don't have the time now."

Richard, who has excellent surgical skills, was operating this morning when one of the older attendings began yelling at him and belittling him over a case, asking in a rage, "Where did you get your training, anyway?" Richard held back the obvious "Here." Last week the same surgeon had Carol in tears when he told her, "You're retarded and you've been that way since you were two!" She is his favorite resident but he becomes verbally abusive in the operating room.

It's been another thirty-six-hour stretch and I'm in a bad state.
Carol told me at three this afternoon that she wants me to work
every Sunday from six A.M. to eight P.M. when I start OB next
month. Our agreement when I took the job was that I'd be able
to leave at five, and although I'll be working six days a week on
OB, I had been looking forward to being home for supper every
night.

"But, Michelle, I'll even let you leave early every afternoon,"
she offered, obviously not understanding why I couldn't do that
—obviously under pressure herself.

"Carol, I'd love to get out early, but I'm not needed at home
in the afternoon the way I am in the evening."

"I'll even give you a whole day off in exchange for those
hours." I knew she needed me and I felt torn, caring about the
work, about Heather, guilty about both.

"Carol, if I work those hours, then I won't see Heather from
Saturday evening until Monday evening, every week. She'll be
asleep when I leave Sunday morning before six, when I get
home Sunday night, and when I leave again Monday morning.
Why don't you make that offer to someone else, three hours for
a whole day? I'm sure the others would love it."

"I can't do that!" was her short reply as she left.

I have such a sense of single motherhood, because if I'm not
there, my child is without a parent. My being able to be home
at suppertime gives a stability to our life because whatever else
happens in the day, I'll be home to take care of it.

A woman in medical school with me had four young children.
She used to get up at five every morning and wake the children
so she could spend time playing with them, since that was the
only time she could count on.

At Heather's day-care center, the other mothers and I, whatever our jobs, shared the feeling that we had already put in a
day's work by the time we got to our job.

•　　　•　　　•

There is a woman on the GYN unit who is seriously ill from an IUD infection. She has been in the hospital for three weeks getting intravenous antibiotics, but signs of infection are still present. We have been doing everything necessary to prevent surgery, which would end her reproductive life.

"You may still have to have surgery," I told her last night because she has been getting worse.

She nodded. "I know that."

Because she seemed so resigned, I told her, "You know, if we do operate, you won't be able to have children."

"But I don't ever want to have children," she said. "I made that decision years ago."

No one had asked her. We had just assumed she wanted to preserve her fertility.

Last night I was upset by all the other women doctors in the hospital—I was struck by how much women have become a part of the system. Years ago when I was working in the hospital for days at a time, it didn't seem so bad because I could tell myself all the others were men and I knew women were different. Now, ten years later, there are many more women, but they are just like the men, taking part in and defending the militaristic training and the insensitive treatment of the patients. Now I feel even more isolated because both men and women comply with the system.

It's not being awake for such long hours that I mind so much; it's the meaninglessness of much of the work. During the day if a patient needs blood, the nursing department gets it from the blood bank, but at night, we have been told, there is no one responsible enough on duty to do that. So at two or three in the morning, only a resident is considered competent enough to go to the lab, compare numbers on the patient's slip and the bag of blood, and bring it back to the patient's room. Half asleep at that hour, I think we are the least capable of the task. It might be all right if we were going home in the morning instead of into the OR for another long day. It would also be easier if those who had been through it weren't saying, "It's good for you. It separates the men from the boys. If you can't take it, you shouldn't be in medicine." I never minded being awake in South Carolina because I was doing useful work, and I don't mind it here when I am doing useful work. It is the senseless, institutionalized "way of doing things" I resent.

I'm so tired after these two days of work without sleep, but tonight I have to go to a gathering of the parents of the children in Heather's class.

Wednesday   *Day 31*

Heather broke down crying as I was leaving for the meeting and asked, "Why are you going out tonight? Why can't you just stay home?"

"Heather, I'm only going out so I can meet the other parents of your school and make it easier for you here," I told her. I stayed and read stories to her until she was feeling better, and then left. It's not like her to act that way. In fact, this has never happened before. Because she so enjoys being with people, a more usual response has been, "When are you going out? I want a baby-sitter."

Among the parents in Heather's class, there are three mothers who are doctors and one who is a medical student. Joan, who will be my chief resident at the end of the year, has a daughter in the same class, but she and her children are away for three months, so the girls have not met each other. She had warned me when I was looking for a place to live, "Don't move as far from the hospital as I have. I don't see my children enough." I don't believe it is the five miles that kept her from them; it's working over a hundred hours a week.

Later

A woman with an infertility problem had a laparoscopy today during which we found adhesions, filmy, spiderweb-like scar tissue that ties organs and structures to each other. As I looked through the laparoscope I could see the purple dye which had been injected through the canula in the cervix and which showed that the Fallopian tubes were open. Nevertheless, the woman will have another operation to remove them because it is presumed that the adhesions are preventing the Fallopian tubes from moving freely.

This evening Barbara came for dinner, partly to meet Heather and partly to see Snuggles, the kitten she had given us. Away from work we relaxed with each other and managed not to talk about work or the people there. Once past her initial shyness, she is open and warm. When she left she said that she now understood why I needed to be home for dinner. As I drove her home she told me that she thought I was very lucky to have a child and that she was jealous. The house is great these days, with Arlene, Gail and Heather. They were all playing music in the living room when I left to take Barbara home.

Thursday   *Day 32*

Fran, a tall graceful woman, was busy setting her coal-black hair and getting ready for a meeting when I stopped by her house on my way home. She took the time, though, to fix me a protein drink, and we talked while she got ready. We talked about how hard it is for women to take care of themselves. She thinks I ought to have something like that drink every morning, and although I agree with her, I know I won't do it. I do such a good job of taking care of Heather. Women seem so often to deny themselves and to nurture others. We worry about balanced meals for our children and then settle for their leftovers as our own.

Before it's too late, I want to get bulbs to plant. I wonder if the house already has bulbs that will come up in the spring. I left many bulbs in the ground when I left the New Jersey house. I especially loved to see the crocuses coming up through the snow.

Bob Carter is a well-known gynecologist with a reputation for charm and a general attitude of "Don't worry about a thing, dearie. I'll take care of you."

Dr. Carter and I were at the sinks scrubbing this morning when he asked, "Can you do a D&C?"

"Sure," I answered.

"Then it's yours to do."

The woman was also having a mole taken off her face, so I did the D&C while he and the plastic surgeon removed the lesion on her face at the other end of the table.

Our next case together was an ovarian cyst and he let me do a lot of it. The woman had been worked up yesterday by Al, a medical student on GYN. She had refused to allow him to do the pelvic exam.

"Okay," he said, "but how about while you are under anesthesia tomorrow?"

"No, I don't want you to examine me then, either. I only want Dr. Carter to examine me."

Today when we were all scrubbing, Dr. Carter told Al to go into the room and examine the woman while she was under anesthesia.

"No. She doesn't want me to," Al said. Dr. Carter kept insisting that it didn't matter whether she had consented, but Al still refused. I admired him for his refusal, but knew the trouble he would be in for what he was doing.

After surgery Carol and I were standing out at the OR desk when Dr. Carter came by to say he was leaving town. Then he leaned over and gave me a pinch on the ass as he left. Containing my rage, I smiled and said, "Have a good trip." Carol and I joked at his having no idea who I really am or how I feel. I was glad to be "in" and accepted, but furious at what that seemed to take.

Yesterday Heather, her friend Megan and I went to the park and flew a new octopus kite with filmy colorful streamers. Heather said it was the "bestest" day ever.

I'm disappointed that I spend so little time reading, but after the intensity of work, I can't pick up a book. I hope to read more on OB, where I imagine there will be more time spent sitting around.

Saturday there was a meeting about women's health care which I didn't attend, but Fran and Laurie brought some of the speakers back to my house for the evening. Maintaining contact with women involved in the politics of women's health care is my antidote to Bob Carter's ass-pinching.

Later

My surgical skills are rapidly improving. This morning I scrubbed on a tubal ligation and then the removal of an ovarian cyst.

The issue of the OB schedule and Carol's wanting me to work a fourteen-hour day every Sunday has me preoccupied. Sometime this morning I told Carol we needed to talk about it, and apparently, I commented that if I had to work those hours I might not stay in the program. I don't remember saying that, but I probably did, since that's how I feel. In one week the thirty-six-hour shifts will be over for a while, and I need that time at home.

Carol and I didn't get to talk until late in the afternoon when she told me she had been in tears after my comment. She felt I didn't care about the program if I could think about leaving, that I didn't care about what it would do to her to be short a person. It was especially strange to hear that I'm needed on the service since mostly I feel that my presence only reminds the others that they are working even more than I.

Starting to cry, I said, "You don't understand the strain I'm under. There's no more of me to go around. All I'm saying is that I've faced the possibility that I may not be able to do all this, that's all. I don't want to leave, but I may not be able to take it."

We were both in tears by then, and I suddenly felt so sorry for her, knowing the strain she is under too. Carol had been chief resident for the past four months, and with the exception of four days in September, she was on call seven days a week, twenty-four hours a day, held responsible for what all the residents did, and subject to Dr. Pierce's rage when anything went wrong.

I didn't want to be fighting with Carol. We were both feeling pushed to our limits. I walked across the room to put my arms around her, and she suddenly stepped back. "You're little!" she said with amazement, standing in front of me.

"Of course I'm little," I told her. "I only seem big," and we both laughed.

Wednesday   Day 38

I kept dreaming last night that I was climbing off elephants and devising systems for climbing off elephants so other people could do it also. I knew it was too far to jump, and I remember that one of the options was to make friends with the elephant so it wouldn't destroy you as you climbed down near its mouth.

Fran and I went wallpaper hunting yesterday. I can't stand the paper in the dining room, but I haven't decided what to put up instead. I debate whether to get vinyl paper, which is easy to put up and care for, or something more formal. The vinyl paper would make it easier to put up Heather's pictures and posters, but I keep finding more formal papers I like. The issue can't be as important as it seems to be, spinning in my head as I try to decide, but I seem stuck with trying to resolve some part of my life via the paper on the dining-room walls.

Heather, Arlene and I had a quiet dinner last night, and then Heather's friends came over and we baked cookies. Now that

Arlene is here I cannot imagine how I ever managed without help in the house. It's so wonderful to come home at night to find that the salad is fixed and that dinner has been planned and is on its way. Even when I cook now I enjoy the nonessential, voluntary nature of what I am doing.

As I drive to work, already a few minutes late, there is a beautiful sunrise in the distance.

Later

Grand Rounds is a weekly formal departmental conference which usually consists of lectures and case presentations. Residents are required to wear white coats and regular clothes as opposed to the grays from the OR.

At Grand Rounds this morning a patient was presented whose current difficulties began six months ago when she had her IUD removed. She had a mild infection at the time, but a week later a tubal ligation was performed in spite of the infection. She has now had three hospitalizations for severe infections and is in danger of dying from infection.

In the second hour of the conference, an anesthesiologist lectured about resuscitation of babies, saying that he found mouth-to-mouth far superior to the bag and mask because he could get a better seal over the nose and mouth with his own mouth. That had been my experience in resuscitating babies: the mask didn't fit well and I could do better without it.

Thursday   *Day 39*

Carol had told me that Dr. Enders, one of the old-timers here, might let me do the hysterectomy today, but after we were gowned he went right to the side of the table, which meant he was doing it. I went to the other side, prepared to assist.

"Knife," he called to the nurse and then cut the woman's skin.

"Snaps," I requested proudly, asking for the little clamps I would use to stop the bleeders as he cut.

Angrily he said, "Marcelle, don't do that. We're not tying them," but in a few minutes, of course we did.

Throughout the surgery, whenever I tried to do something, it was wrong, but when I didn't do anything, that was wrong too. When I saw a bleeder and said something to him, since I no longer spontaneously did anything, he would snap at me, "I have eyes. I can see!" But when I was quiet, he asked, "Why aren't you doing something to help here? Want her to bleed to death?"

I had looked forward to the surgery this morning, practicing knots and reading last night at home. Dr. Enders insists on calling me Marcelle too, which bugs me.

Tomorrow I'm on for twenty-four hours, then again on Sunday for another twenty-four, and then Tuesday I begin three months of OB. Beth, who will be on OB at night, has agreed to come in early Sunday evening in exchange for other time off. I'll be working six days a week, but I'll be home for dinner every night. With only six weeks behind me, I am sometimes overwhelmed by what I have committed myself to doing. I wonder how long I will last.

Saturday   *Day 41*

Much of the last twenty-four hours has been enjoyable, in spite of only two hours' sleep, because the work was challenging, and I was learning.

In the OR yesterday morning I put on my first set of Fallope rings, finding it easy to see what I was doing. Then I scrubbed on a myomectomy with Dr. Ingle, another one of the old-timers here; he is a skilled surgeon, but reticent to say much. He asked me to dictate the operative notes when we were through, so I wished he had been open to more questions about what we were doing.

Busy in the OR until late in the afternoon, I had little time on the floor before I was called back for emergency surgery on a woman with an ectopic pregnancy. We did laparoscopy first, trying to be certain what she had, but when we saw the bleeding in her pelvis we opened her up, located the ruptured ectopic pregnancy and removed the Fallopian tube. Charlie, the chief for the night, did most of the surgery, but he let me close the abdomen. He talked about what he was doing as he worked, so I learned a great deal. He's a really nice guy who cares about his patients and about those of us who work with him.

Around midnight I was called to the emergency room to see a woman with a severe pelvic infection and an IUD still in place. I removed the IUD and began giving her antibiotics. The IUD is so dangerous, causing infections and infertility, and increasing the incidence of ectopic pregnancy because of infections and subsequent damage to the Fallopian tubes.

The rest of the night was spent taking care of the woman on whom Dr. Enders and I did the hysterectomy. Her past history of severe kidney disease had caused me to worry about her having surgery, especially since it was for fibroids, relatively harmless, though they were giving her pain. She now has a life-threatening infection following the surgery. I'm bothered by the number of life-threatening infections I am seeing.

Monday   *Day 43*

It's been a long twenty-six hours, but some of the time was actually pleasurable. The hours after midnight are the painful ones.

Yesterday morning after rounds, I relaxed and took time to think about my patients, plan for their care for the day, and leave good summarizing notes on their charts for the next group of residents.

A woman came into the emergency room with pelvic pain. It was discovered in surgery to be a ruptured ovarian cyst, which we removed. The anesthesiology resident had a lot of trouble getting the needle into the woman's spine and she gave the impression that she didn't care. Eventually her supervisor arrived and placed the needle, but then the resident spilled the medication on the floor. Finally the anesthesiologist said we could begin.

"Knife," called the surgeon, and taking the scalpel in his hand, made one long incision. The woman screamed in pain, blood appeared on her skin, and the anesthesiologist quickly put her under with general anesthesia. It had taken two hours to begin.

An abortion is the expulsion of a nonviable fetus. In lay language, abortion usually refers to removal of the fetus through medical intervention, while miscarriage is used to denote a spontaneous loss of a fetus. However, in medicine, the term abortion includes all fetal loss.

I did two D&Cs today for incomplete abortions. In these situations a woman has placental or other tissue left and is usually bleeding. Then another woman came into the emergency room with a threatened abortion, cramping and bleeding, and she passed the fetus this morning. Early this morning I admitted another woman having an incomplete abortion, and she will have her D&C this morning.

Last night at six, Heather, Arlene and Gail stopped by the hospital on their way to the movies and brought supper for me. I had prepared a CARE package for Heather in case I couldn't get out of the OR, containing a hair brush, toothbrush, Band-Aids and skin cream I had collected from the patient supplies cabinet. I was able to see them, though, and we had a short visit in the lobby before they went off to the movies.

Tomorrow morning I begin obstetrics, the part of the program I especially came here for. I worry about what it will be like to be a part of the highly technological childbirth practiced in the hospital. I want to know the technology, to understand it and be able to use it when necessary.

Nationally the Caesarean section has become epidemic, with some hospitals reporting as much as 40 to 50 percent incidence. I want to be able to do my own Caesareans, and not have to turn over women in trouble to doctors whose childbirth philosophies may be so different from mine or that of the woman. It is learning the obstetrics that brought me to Doctors Hospital.

Chapter Four

The C-Section

There is a natural opening in a pregnant woman—the vagina—through which a baby can usually pass. When babies are born this way, there is not much for a physician to do except watch. However, when the physician needs to get the baby out through the woman's abdomen, s/he can take it out using knives, scissors, clamps, needles and metal clips to cut through the abdomen and through the uterus. The Caesarean section is a major surgical operation.

The woman coming into the hospital for an elective—i.e., planned, nonemergency—section is admitted early the day before so she can have a work-up, be seen by anesthesia, have lab tests, etc. She is usually healthy and well prepared for what will happen to her. Doctors seem better able to tell a woman about a forthcoming Caesarean section than a vaginal delivery. The type of anesthesia has usually been decided, as well as whether the incision, and thus the resulting scar, will be vertical, from the bellybutton to the pubic bone, or along the pubic hairline in the "bikini cut." The type of anesthesia generally determines whether the husband will be allowed to stay in the OR, since in most hospitals he cannot be present if she has general anesthesia.

The explanation usually given for this policy is that the man's presence is only justified if his wife is awake and they can share the experience. Anesthesiologists generally do not like to have visitors in the operating room. Since they have only a transient relationship with the patient, they have less investment in meeting her needs for a support person. The obstetrician, on the other hand, often has an ongoing relationship with the woman and wants her to be satisfied with her birth experience.

Examining the woman's abdomen as part of the H&P, I first feel the general position of the baby and then listen with the stethoscope. In addition to the heartbeat, the baby can be heard as well as felt as it kicks and rolls, making bulges, arranging space, seeking a slightly more comfortable position, like someone under a deep layer of covers. Handing the stethoscope to the mother, I help her listen, sometimes commenting on what the baby is doing or trying to do.

Babies must feel good when they kick. There is a freedom and then a resistance, the freedom of weightlessness, then the gentle resistance of fluid giving way before moving limbs, and then the firmer resistance of the uterine walls. They are like swimmers in a pool who, reaching the end of the lane, twist their bodies around and kick off again. The baby in utero is never untouched, never in a void. There's always the fluid passing, there are always the walls to be felt with feet, knees, fists, head.

There are sounds inside, too, of water moving, of the baby's own intestinal rumblings, of the mother's heart, the mother's intestinal rumblings, the mother's voice. There are sensations of swallowing, of urinating, of pressure changes, of tightness, of movement. In a Caesarean birth the baby has little warning that its peaceful world will change. Without the preparation of labor, birth is abrupt.

In the morning the woman is wheeled on a stretcher to the L&D (Labor and Delivery) suite, and then to the delivery room, which doubles as a section room. For epidural anesthesia, the woman is placed on the operating table on her left side. She is told to curl into a fetal-like position to allow a needle to be inserted between the vertebrae of her curved spine. When the needle is withdrawn, leaving a tube in the spine, the woman is placed flat on her back and the table temporarily tilted slightly to lower her head in order to establish a level of anesthesia that is high enough to make the woman's abdomen numb, but won't affect her ability to breathe. There is only a fine margin of both safety and comfort: if the level is too low, she will have pain during the surgery; if it is too high, she will have difficulty breathing and will require mechanical assistance. The woman's bladder is next catheterized and the tube left in the bladder to keep urine draining. During the surgery the bladder is cut away from the surface of the uterus as there is a greater risk of perforating or cutting into it if it is full.

Preparation of the surgical site consists of scrubbing and draping the abdomen, with only that portion to be cut left exposed. It is similar to any other surgical preparation except for the inhibited discussion if the woman is awake.

I had been wondering why I always got so covered with blood and amniotic fluid during a Caesarean section, while the surgeon would come out so much cleaner. I would be soaked through my gown, my greens and my underwear. It was finally explained to me: "The table is tilted slightly so the blood and fluid run onto the assistant and not onto the surgeon."

As soon as the woman is draped, the anesthesiologist tilts the table to one side and signals for the surgeon to begin. The surgeon takes a scalpel from the nurse and with one strong and definite motion creates a crescent-shaped incision along the woman's pubic hairline. As the skin is cut, the subcutaneous tissue bulges upward as though it had been straining to get through all the time. Within moments this fatty tissue, interconnected by thin transparent fibers, becomes dotted and then covered with blood that oozes out of tiny vessels. With scalpel and forceps—delicate tweezers—the surgeon cuts deeper beneath the subcutaneous tissue, to a thick layer of fibrous tissue that holds the abdominal organs and muscles of the abdominal wall in place. Once reached, this fibrous layer is incised and cut along the lines of the original surface incision while the muscles adhering to this tissue are scraped off and pushed out of the way. The uterus is now visible under the peritoneum, a layer of thin tissue, looking like Saran Wrap, which covers most of the internal organs and which, when inflamed, produces peritonitis. The peritoneum is lifted away from the uterus and an incision is made in it, leaving the uterus and bladder easily accessible. The bladder is peeled away from the uterus, for the baby will be taken out through an incision in the uterus underneath where the bladder usually lies. When a Caesarean is done as an emergency procedure and speed is essential, the bladder is not removed and instead the incision is made much higher in the uterus. This produces weaker scar tissue and greater chance of rupture during a subsequent pregnancy and labor.

The uterus of the pregnant woman is large, smooth and glistening. Shaped like a huge pear, the top and sides are thick and muscular, the lower end thin and flexible. With short careful strokes of a knife, a small incision is made through the thinner segment. Special care is taken not to cut the baby or the membranes surrounding the baby which, if still intact, now bulge through the tiny hole in the uterus. The room becomes silent: the quiet presence of the baby about to be born causes time suddenly to stop.

The obstetrician extends the initial cut either by putting two index fingers into the small incision and ripping the uterus open or by using blunt-ended scissors and cutting in two directions away from the initial incision. If the membranes are still intact, they are now punctured with toothed forceps, and the fluid spills out onto the table. In the normal position, the baby's head is down and under the incision, so the obstetrician places one hand inside the uterus, under the baby's head, and with the other hand exerts pressure on the upper end of the uterus to push the baby through the abdominal incision. The assistant also uses force now to help push the baby out. Once the baby's head is out, the throat is immediately suctioned with a small ear syringe, and then the shoulders and rest of the body are eased out. Held in the air, the baby usually begins to cry. The cord is clamped and the baby handed over to a nurse holding a warmed towel. Sometimes, en route to the nurse, the infant is momentarily held over the woman's head with its genitals facing down into the mother's face, as she is told, "Look, it's a boy/girl!" The assumption is always made that the woman wants most to know and see the sex of her child. For many women, including those delivering vaginally, this is all they see of their babies at the time of delivery.

The rest of the surgery is more difficult for the woman. There is more pain and women often vomit and complain of difficult breathing as we handle their organs and repair the damage. This period may also be more difficult because there is no longer the anticipation of waiting to see the baby born. Sometimes the woman is given sedation for the rest of the surgery.

The placenta separates from or is peeled off the inside of the uterus. Then, since the uterine attachments are all at the lower end, near the cervix, the body of the uterus can be brought out of the abdominal cavity and rested on the outside of the woman's abdomen, thus adding both visibility and room in which to work.

With large circular needles and thick thread a combination of running and individual stitches is used to sew closed the hole in the uterus. A drug called pitocin is added to the woman's IV to help the uterus contract and to decrease the bleeding. Small sutures are used to tie and retie bleeding blood vessels. The "gutters," spaces in the abdominal cavity, are cleared of blood and fluid. The uterus is then placed back in the abdominal cavity. The bladder is sewn back onto the surface of the uterus, and then finally the peritoneum is closed. Now sponges are counted to be sure none have been left inside the abdominal cavity, and then the closure of the abdominal wall begins.

Muscles overlying the peritoneum are pushed back in place, and are sometimes sewn with loose stitches. Fascia, the thick fibrous layer, is the most important one, since it holds all the abdominal organs inside and keeps them from coming through the incision, especially if the woman coughs or sneezes. Therefore this layer is closed with heavy thread and many individual stitches so that, even if a thread breaks, the stitches won't all come out. The subcutaneous tissue, most of which is fat, is closed in loose stitches that mainly close any air spaces which might become sites for infection. Skin, the final layer, is closed with either silk or nylon thread or metal staples. The appearance of the final scar is generally considered important, since many people judge whether a surgeon is good or not by the scar's appearance.

A dry bandage is placed over the woman's incision and then taped to her skin. The drapes are removed. A baby has been born.

MODERN CHILDBIRTH

Childbirth in a hospital is both conducted and described as a technological event. As a resident at Doctors Hospital I write on a chart: "NSD [normal spontaneous delivery] from ROA [right occiput anterior] over ML Epis. [midline episiotomy] of male infant, Apgar 9/10. EBL [estimated blood loss] 50 cc., repair 3-0 chromic sutures. Mother to RR [recovery room] good condition. Infant to nursery." I sign that note illegibly, ashamed to "take credit" for that delivery.

That is the standard way of describing the more common vaginal birth. The position (ROA in this case) refers to the relationship of the baby's head to the mother's pelvis. Its importance is primarily related to the use of forceps when it is critical to know the position of the head in order to correctly apply the blades of the forceps. The episiotomy—the cutting of the perineum of the woman to increase the size of the vaginal opening through which the baby passes—is considered by most physicians to be part of a normal delivery.

The Apgar score, taught early in medical school, is a standardized set of criteria by which one rates the condition of the baby at one minute and then at five minutes. One asks a colleague, or sometimes even the mother, "How was the baby?" and is told, "The Apgar was _____." Scores are added up from the following table.

	2	1	0
heart rate	over 100	below 100	absent
breathing and crying	prompt, lusty	slow, irregular	no breathing, 1–2 gasps
reflex irritability (response to slap on foot or catheter in nose or throat)	vigorous cry	grimace	no response
muscle tone	active motion	some flexion of extremities	flaccid
color	completely pink	body pink, extremities blue	blue, pale

A top score is obviously 10. Most babies have Apgar scores between 7 and 9 at one minute, and 8 and 10 at five minutes. Those in severe distress are between 0 and 3. A baby with a high Apgar looks good, one with a low one looks bad.

The Apgar is a research tool. If we study ten thousand babies with an Apgar of 3, for ten years, we have certain information that can usually be summed up as: "Babies who are ill at birth often have a hard time in life." The Apgar tells us little, however, about any particular baby's prognosis and nothing about who that person is going to be and how that new person's life will be lived.

What do we need to know about a birth? What are we missing when we score a baby by heartbeats per minute? What are the questions we should be asking as we try to describe the emergence of one human being out of the body of another?

Was there awe?
Do those in the room feel close to each other and the baby?
Does this baby look healthy?
Does this baby feel welcomed into the world?
Does the baby make eye contact?
Is the baby curious?
Does the baby respond to touch, to voice, to being held?
What is the mother's mood? Happy? Depressed? Frightened?
What is the baby's mood? Happy? Depressed? Frightened?
Was the baby smiling in the birth canal?
Does this mother feel good about herself after this birth?
Is the mother ready to move on to the next phase of their
   relationship, whether that is together or apart?
Was love present?

We listen for a new baby's crying so we don't have to look at it. A baby doesn't have to be crying for us to know it is healthy. Hold a new baby. It makes eye contact. It breathes. It sighs. The baby has color. Lift it in your arms and feel whether it has good tone or poor, strong limbs or limp ones. The baby does not have to be on a cold table to have its condition measured. What do we lose by being kind to a baby who has just been born?

Babies look serene as they are being born. I do not believe they have just been through trauma. When a baby has been hurt or frightened, it cries and is difficult to console. Babies coming out of their mothers do not cry. There is a myth shared by doctors and mothers that a baby suffers during its passage through the woman's pelvis. True, we, as adults, would find it excruciating, trying to squeeze through, but the baby is soft and pliable—even its skull is soft. When it comes out of the vagina, it bears no signs of having suffered yet. A baby cries when it hits air, when it is suspended by its feet, when its cord is cut and it must gasp for air, when it is overwhelmed by loud sound and bright lights.

•   •   •

Jeremy is born after fourteen hours of his mother's labor at home in New Jersey. She is kneeling, pushing him out and down between her legs. As the baby's head emerges, his lips are pursed, his eyes squeezed closed. Another push brings him out past his bellybutton, when he opens his eyes and seems quietly to be waiting to see what will happen next. His body out, I suction mucus from his mouth and he protests with short cries. The cord begins to close off his blood supply, so he takes a sudden gasp for air, and finding that successful, breathes more easily. I pass him through his mother's legs to her waiting hands, but in the awkwardness of the transfer, he begins to cry. She takes him to her chest and rocking him in her arms, is able to soothe him.

He is peaceful again, eyes open, beginning to seek out form. I do not believe he has just been through a terrible ordeal.

When I was in medical school, the ward patients in labor received little or no pain relief, while the private patients were given scopolamine, a drug that wiped out the memory of the labor and birth. Many women loved it and would say, "My doctor was wonderful. He gave me a shot to put me out as soon as I came to the hospital. I never felt a thing." Those women weren't put out, but they didn't remember what had happened to them—or at least not consciously. When these women thought they were "out" they were awake and screaming. Made crazy from the drug, they fought; they growled like animals. They had to be restrained, tied by hands and feet to the corners of the bed (with straps padded with lamb's wool so there would be no injury, no telltale marks) or they would run screaming down the halls. Screaming obscenities, they bit, they wept, behaving in ways that would have produced shame and humiliation had they been aware. Doctors and nurses, looking at such behavior induced by the drug they had administered, felt justified in treating the women as crazy wild animals to be tied, ordered, slapped, yelled at, gagged.

When it is all over, the mother thanks the doctor. She sends her friends to him, saying, "It was wonderful. I never felt a thing."

The doctor in the hospital calls out to the woman strapped to the delivery table, "It's a boy." The mother must wait to be told the sex of her child. At one of my first home births, the woman was standing up, the only position she was comfortable in. Trying to be where I could best take care of the baby as it came out and down between her legs, I lay on the floor under her, facing upward between her legs. As the baby's head came out facing backward, its buttocks slid forward between the woman's legs and in front of her. She called out, "My son! My son!" telling us the sex of her child.

When I attended home births I carried no pain medications: I told the women they would have to go to the hospital if they needed such medication, because all the drugs have some depressive effects on the babies. Mothers given drugs that derange them or do them physical damage are no better off. An angry obstetrician confronted me once at a meeting in New Jersey, where, shouting across a table which separated us, he asked, "But, Dr. Harrison, what do you do when a woman is in pain?" He was shaking his fist, accusing me of cruelty and inhumanity.

"When a woman is in pain, I put my arms around her and I hold her," I said.

I understood why he was upset. Any decent person, confronted with a woman in pain, of course wants to give her relief. The problem is that in our society, one way to say "help me" is "give me a drug." That "relief" they are seeking, that drug the physician is administering, can be very harmful to the woman and to her child.

I was trying to say that there are alternative responses to the woman's cry for help. Touch, a soothing voice, eye contact, even just the physician's supportive presence in the room can bring the woman safely through her pain.

There was a vivid example of this when a nurse I knew was giving birth at home. As soon as I arrived at her house she began screaming, "Michelle, give me something. Put me out! I can't stand it!"

"I don't have anything, you know that," I said as I sat down on the bed, my arm around her shoulder.

"Can't you give me something?" she implored.

Moved by the pain in her voice and eyes, I tried to communicate my wish to help her. "If you really can't take it, let's go to the hospital. It's okay, I'll take you in."

She said she didn't want to go and went on to deliver within the hour.

Afterward she told me, "It was good to know I could beg for anything, and you *couldn't* give it to me. It was safe to scream because I knew you didn't carry drugs and wouldn't sedate me."

Sometimes a woman screams to make the pain go away, not to be drugged.

I am not opposed to drugs on principle, but there is no painless childbirth because there is no medication that does not also interfere with the mother and/or the child. Some of that damage we know, and some we don't because we do not look. In the hospital I would not deny relief to a woman who wants it, but her decision should be made on the basis of valid information, including the risks both to herself or her child. It is not a choice for anyone else to make. Our need to "do something" to "quiet her," can even result in her being pressured to accept medication. Often the drug doesn't take the pain away. It only makes the woman less able to cope with it, making her drowsy or loosening her control of herself.

Scopolamine is not used at Doctors Hospital, where childbirth is said to be modern, technological and humane. The woman doesn't need amnesia because she is told that hers is the finest childbirth experience available, and if it doesn't seem that way to her, she assumes it's her own fault. If she is among the 33 percent of women who have a Caesarean at this hospital, then she is made to feel thankful she is living in this age of technology so her baby could be "saved."

Integral to modern technological childbirth is the fetal monitor, which is applied either externally around the mother's abdomen or internally by means of a metal electrode that is screwed into the scalp of the baby still in utero. The screw on the end of the monitor is shaped like the end of a corkscrew, and as it is twisted, it pierces the baby's scalp and hooks 1 to 2 millimeters into the skin. The external monitor uses ultrasound waves to record the heartbeat, although ultrasound has never been proven safe for babies. In experimental studies, ultrasound has been found to have effects similar to x-rays. The monitor console, a machine about the size of a portable dishwasher, is on wheels so it can be brought to the bedside. Long wires then connect the machine either to the internal or external attachments to mother and/or baby. Across the top of the machine is a window through which graph paper travels while a black needle marks each beat of the baby's heart. Additional leads can be used to measure pressure in the uterus or timing of contractions.

The amplified fetal heartbeat sounds like galloping horses, so with two or three monitors going in a room, the sound is one of a galloping herd. In the hall, the sounds of different monitors in different rooms fuse into a roar of childbirth. Frequently there are also the intermittent commands to the women, "Push! Push!," reminiscent of stampedes and posse chases in the old Westerns. Both the sound of the galloping and the vision of the needle traveling across the paper, making a blip with each heartbeat, are hypnotic, often giving one the illusion that the machines are keeping the baby's heart beating.

At Doctors Hospital I learned to screw a monitor lead into the scalp of a baby not yet born. Is the baby still smiling? Was the baby smiling before I screwed the electrical lead into its head? Was the baby frightened? Is this baby curious anymore? Does this baby still want to be with us? What have we taught this new person about what life is like?

At Doctors Hospital I attached the woman to the monitor, and after that, no one looked at her anymore. Held in place by the leads around her abdomen and coming out of her vagina, the woman looked over at the TV-like screen displaying the heartbeat tracings. No one held the woman's hand. Childbirth had become a science.

Still wanting to know more about that science and those truths promised by the new technology, I had sought further training. For a long time I believed my presence in the hospital —on the "inside"—could make a difference, that my different perspective could affect the way in which women were treated.

Doctors Hospital was known both for its humane modern childbirth practices and its technical sophistication. From this hospital, affiliated with one of the world's leading educational institutions, originated many of the country's standards for hospital obstetrics. The doctors who taught me also created the truths taught elsewhere. I had come to Mecca, but I was unprepared for the dehumanized process—birth—I found there.

LABOR AND DELIVERY (L&D)

The L&D suite was an enclosed area in which a woman spent the duration of her labor, delivery and recovery. There were three beds in each of three labor rooms, but when they were full, the recovery room and hallways were also used for laboring women. Through heavy gray doors were the four delivery rooms, two of which were also equipped for doing Caesarean sections.

Outside the L&D suite was a converted single patient room referred to as the Alternative Birth Service, or ABS. The room was decorated with curtains, a picture on the wall, a plant on the sill, and drapes which hid all the obstetrical equipment. A single stretcherlike bed dominated the room with space enough for one chair on either side. Because the room was outside L&D it was necessary to have a nurse available to stay in the room when a woman was laboring. A woman planning to use the room had to be at "low risk," meaning no complications were expected. The arrangements had to have been made in advance of labor, her doctor or midwife had to have approved her use of the room, and there had to be available nursing personnel at the time the woman was admitted in labor.

Women who moved to ABS, after being admitted to L&D until good labor was certain, often experienced a slowing or cessation of their labor. This may have been related to the "specialness" of the room, the need for constant nursing personnel, and the fear of how far they were from the full technology available on L&D.

There was also a doctors' lounge, a large sparse room with an x-ray-viewing box, a TV, some chairs, a small desk, and lockers for the attendings. The closet rarely had any hangers, so clothes were usually folded and left on the floor. A door at the far end of the lounge led to a bathroom and then to a second small room with two beds, also to be used only by attendings. I had heard that one of the attendings had occasionally let his children sleep there, so I hoped in an emergency I could do the same.

A coffee room outside the labor rooms was the main place for congregating, especially for the nurses, who had no lounge.

The only place in which to be alone in the area was a long linen and supply closet where, even with the door open, one could hide unnoticed behind the racks of supplies. Carol showed me the closet one day during my first week on OB, saying that she and Jackie and Joan had named it the "crying closet." It was at the window of that closet, looking down at the streets, that Carol told me of the prevalent talk of suicide among the women residents.

Carol, Jackie and Joan had all come to OB wanting to change the way that women were treated. For women physicians with such a perspective, the daily assault on female patients they have to watch and take part in is painful, confusing and isolating. It is often difficult for women to make the transition that is required of them: from identifying with a sister to seeing her impersonally, as a patient. Unfortunately, most often they do not make the transition, and the attitudes of female obstetricians and gynecologists is indistinguishable from that of their male colleagues.

•   •   •

Richard was my chief on obstetrics. Hoping we could make a fresh start in working together, I went to him a few days before we started OB and asked how I could best prepare. He showed me how to fill out all the data sheets for each delivery—the only time he willingly taught me anything. I kept trying to be nice to Richard, thinking he wouldn't be so awful if he knew me better.

Richard was the most competitive person I met at DH. He was a loner who was putting in his time until the following year when he would begin a special GYN surgical fellowship. Cancer was his primary interest; he could tolerate obstetrics only because, as he said, "Childbirth is a surgical procedure."

John was the first-year resident who worked the day OB shift with me. Twenty-five years old and single, he flirted with the nurses and could often be overheard asking some of the younger attendings to arrange dates for him. John would say of *his* patients, "I like *my girls* to stay on the thinner side during pregnancy."

John resented my working part-time. When I wasn't there he complained that he had too much work to do, but when I was there he said he didn't get enough deliveries. It seems terrible that we were the people who were supposed to be taking care of women having babies. We weren't in any shape to take part in a happy event. We cried, we fought about deliveries, we competed, we dumped on each other, we argued procedures.

Tuesday morning   *Day 44*

I am living in two worlds. Fran and Laurie and Gail are using my den to work on some resource booklets on women's health. Last night I went to sleep to the sound of Fran's typing. The sound of other people carrying on was comforting for me. It erases my own sense of isolation. At home I am in the world of women, self-care, consumer control; I am living and working with people who every day challenge the health-care system, especially as it treats women.

I drive the five miles to the hospital, where the doctor's word is law, the patient's proper attitude is submission. Somewhere between these two worlds I search for a truth, a balance, and a place for myself.

Fran has been very receptive to my thoughts and feelings about abortion. I believe in the right of a woman to have an abortion, but doing them is difficult for me. When I was in medical school and abortions were illegal, we would daily treat women who were critically ill from attempted illegal abortions. It was not unusual for such a woman to die as a result of infection. Even five years ago, when I was teaching at the medical school, I realized that students were graduating without ever seeing the catastrophic results of illegally induced abortions. It's like an epidemic disease that has been irradicated, but which will surely return if the legislation is changed again and abortions become illegal.

Because Fran is so involved in protecting the rights of women to have abortions, I hesitated for a while to share with her how painful it was to do them. Her sympathetic response was a surprise.

After the day

I met Richard in the parking lot when I got to work and he told me to meet him on 3W, a floor of about twenty to twenty-five postpartum patients. I waited there for fifteen minutes, uncertain about what I was supposed to do. I began looking through charts and then making rounds on the patients, which is what the nurse said the previous residents did. When Richard came to 3W at twenty to eight, I tried to ask him some questions about the wound on a patient I'd seen. He said he'd look at her. I tried to go with him but he told me to continue rounds. By the time I finished seeing the next woman he was gone and had left a note saying "She was okay," and I couldn't ask him any questions.

I was in the middle of taking out sutures from a Caesarean incision when the nurse came by and said, "It's five after eight and Richard wants you on L&D immediately." I finished taking out the stitches and went up to L&D to find Richard angry that

I hadn't been there at eight. He said I must be on L&D at eight even if I have not finished rounds, but that I was really supposed to finish rounds on those twenty-odd women before eight.

I tried to find out such details as who I was to see, who was to be discharged, what kind of responsibility I had for which patients, but Richard was of no help. I asked him about service patients, those without attendings, and he said there were none. I protested that I had seen one chart, so there must be one such patient on the floor. He answered, "I forgot." The truth is that if the service patient doesn't get seen by a resident, she gets no care.

Later in the day I went back to 3W and took as much time as I needed. One woman remarked with obvious pleasure about how much time I was taking with her and I said, "I have the luxury to do that today; by tomorrow I will have been told I can't." Of course that is what happened later in the day; Richard told me I couldn't spend so much time with patients.

I spent some time talking with Kara, a teen-ager who had a baby two days ago, and Janie, the older sister with whom she lives. Kara is planning to enter the Service, and Janie, who is still nursing her own ten-month-old, is nursing her baby for her, leaving Kara feeling somewhat left out of the care of her new baby. Last night Janie was unable to come in, and Kara pumped her own breast to put the milk in a bottle for her baby. I suggested to both of them that Kara might want to nurse the baby with her sister and that they might even enjoy trading nursing times with both babies. Kara had been told that she either had to nurse all the time or not nurse at all. The two sisters and I talked about ways they could share the mothering of Kara's baby, even though Kara would be leaving after six months. I enjoyed the time I spent with them, aware that I would not often have the opportunity to speak with patients so openly or so thoroughly.

Richard showed me how circumcisions are done here, since residents on OB do them. We went to the newborn nursery, where he took the baby into the treatment room, put him in a large molded plastic frame with Velcro straps for the baby's body, arms and legs. He put a steel clamp on the baby's penis, but then left the room to take a phone call and was gone for three or four minutes. Finding myself alone in the room with the baby, I began to pat him gently and sing to him. I sang the lullaby I had sung to my niece Abigail when she was just a few hours old and I was with her in the newborn nursery.

My first delivery at DH was with Dr. Hilda Cameron, an attending I hadn't met until I was taking care of her laboring patient. I told her I was new here, but I don't think she heard me. Just before the delivery I took the woman back to the delivery room and had her prepped and draped by the time Hilda got there.

"I think you should do the episiotomy on the next contraction," she told me.

I was not used to doing episiotomies, since at home births I had learned to deliver babies without cutting the perineum. I asked her, "Do you routinely do episiotomies?" She had just commented on how much room there was for the baby, since the woman had a loose perineum, so I had hoped we might leave it alone.

She responded brusquely, "Nothing is routine in obstetrics. Now do the episiotomy."

My hand was shaking as I took the scissors and tried to make a very small cut.

"Deeper! Deeper!" she said and then angrily took the scissors from my hand and made a large cut in the woman's perineum and extended the cut into the vagina. We delivered the baby on the next contraction.

"It's a girl!" Hilda called out, and then I looked and said, "No, it's a boy," and she corrected herself. Then she began to sew. The woman was having some pain, although she had been given epidural anesthesia and should have been okay. The anesthesiologist increased the dosage, and finally the woman was numb. Hilda was thinking about giving her Demerol intravenously for the pain and I kept thinking about how drowsy the woman would then be.

The child was blue for a short while, but it cried a lot and seemed healthy. The woman kept looking over at the baby and watching him cry and trying to talk to her baby across the room.

Although I came here to learn the hospital way of delivery, I am opposed to the routine performance of episiotomies on women. The usual reasons given for doing them are: to prevent excessive stretching of the muscles by the baby pushing through, which would result in weakened support for the bladder. That this results has never been proven. A second reason for episiotomies is to maintain vaginal tightness, presumably for the pleasure of a future sex partner. That may in fact be true, but I'm not sure it warrants a surgical procedure, since there are exercises that tighten the pelvic muscles again.

Think of the episiotomy this way: if you hold a piece of cloth at two corners and attempt to tear it by pulling at the two ends, it will rarely rip. However, if a small cut is made in the center, then pulling at the ends easily rips the cloth. Doing an episiotomy is analogous, and sometimes results in tears that extend into the rectum. Physicians argue that this "clean" tear is more easily repaired than the ragged one that occurs when a woman tears without the cut. My experience has been that the small tears that sometimes occur without episiotomy are easy to stitch and less bothersome to the woman.

Episiotomies, once repaired, are often debilitating and are the source of much pain in the immediate postpartum period, at a time when a woman might most want mobility in taking care of her newborn. Whether a woman will have one done is a frequent source of anxiety during pregnancy.

My final objection is that the woman is rarely given a choice in the matter.

Later in the day John put his first internal monitor lead into a baby's scalp. The patient was a woman in her late twenties who spoke some English but with a heavy accent. Each time the curtain around her bed was opened, she would signal for someone to close it. First John ruptured the membranes, and then with the woman's legs apart, he put his hand in her vagina and screwed the electrode into the baby's head. The baby's heart rate fell and everyone worried for a few minutes, but then it returned to normal.

Present in the room, besides the patient, were: her husband, two nurses, myself; John, Richard—who was instructing John—and some student nurses. There are some old pictures around of medicine in history, in which you can see leeches being applied, or bloodletting. The paintings have an aura of foreboding about them, fear of what is happening. I thought about those pictures and suddenly wondered what had changed. The technology is different, but the crowd of people standing around the bed is the same. The only difference is that now women are among those dispensing the technology. I wanted to cry for this woman, I wanted to tell her to go home and have her baby at home without wires in its head.

Later the woman began to want to push, although she was only eight centimeters dilated. The nurses called for her attending, who was not available, and I agreed to take a look at her. She was about at that stage when, during a home birth, I would have allowed her to start gently pushing. Instead she had the nurses standing there saying "Don't push! Don't push!" and scolding her. One nurse said, "If you push, you will hurt the baby." I felt helpless.

The woman continued to want to push. Richard was located and came to check her. By then she was nine centimeters, and then quickly fully dilated. By this time, though, it was strange because she no longer seemed to have the same urge to push, and she was no longer in control of herself or able to respond to what was happening in her body. When she was told to push she had difficulty. It was sad because she had been so sure before and had been responding so strongly to what her body wanted her to do. Now she was also forced to lie on her back, rather than on her side, in order to push. I kept thinking of the women who delivered at home squatting, and on their knees, or on their sides.

Chapter Five

HOME/HOSPITAL BIRTH

At the end of the first day on OB, I wondered with panic what I had done in coming there. I had expected that what I would learn would be different from what I had been doing. What I hadn't considered was how different it would feel. It was as though these two worlds of birthing that I knew could not exist at the same time: as if the atmosphere and the power of the hospital was so overwhelming, it allowed only one definition of reality, one possibility of what could happen.

Images of the women I had delivered at home came to me and were quickly replaced by the overhanging lights of the delivery rooms; the silence of a woman laboring at home was lost in the noise of the galloping monitors and the commanding voices.

What was a home birth, that other experience I had known?

ONE HOME BIRTH: ONE DAY LAST YEAR

Marie called this afternoon to say she was having irregular contractions and she thinks she may be going into labor. She's letting me know early so I can think about which appointments I may have to cancel. It is a Saturday afternoon early in summer.

Heather is off with friends and I call to be sure she can stay with them for the night in case Marie is really in labor.

I think about Marie and this forthcoming birth. I begin to feel the tension of anticipation. I sense that this will be the day. There are times my own menstrual cycle seems attuned to the births ahead. At once I feel a part of the process, a witness, participant, recorder.

Marie doesn't yet need me at the house. Her husband is with her and they will call me when they need me to be there. This is her second pregnancy, but her first birth at home.

For me the hours before a birth are long: I am already absorbed in thinking about and preparing myself for this birth, so it is difficult for me to do anything that requires my full attention. I go to a pool near my home, a place where I feel most peacefully alone. It is a strain always to be on call, always to have to respond to someone else's need. When I am in the middle of the pool, swimming long laps, I know I have until I reach the end of the lane before I can be paged. It may only be another thirty seconds, but that time is mine.

I swim until my tiredness passes, and from then on I feel I can swim indefinitely. Each lap of the pool seems to give me strength to store up for what is coming. It is hard work to deliver babies, especially at home. I use everything I have— memory, skill, intuition—as well as everything I sense. I must do all that in an atmosphere where inattention can have disastrous effects on this mother, this baby, on me personally and on the general acceptance of home birth.

Swimming laps, I recall a visit I made earlier to Marie and Alex at home, as I do with each home-birth woman in the latter part of her pregnancy. Marie's house surprised me when I first got there. It was a large white Colonial, in a community of well-landscaped suburban homes. Elegantly furnished, it had a living room of champagne-colored carpeting and a white upholstered sofa. I thought, She's got one child already, she's expecting a second—and she has white furniture.

We had set the visit for early evening so Alex, a banker, could be home. We sat in the living room, talking and drinking lemonade. From time to time Liza, their three-year-old, would amble through, say hello, play and move on. The carpet remained champagne, the sofa white.

Marie and Alex told me they wanted to have their baby at home because they wanted control over their environment— including no drugs. If something went wrong, they wanted to be part of any decisions that were made. Alex said, "In the hospital as soon as something is slightly off, they take over completely. They use all their guns."

"Last time they gave me a needle in my back and I never felt the rest. I want to experience childbirth. I want to know what it is like and I want to be able to get through it" was Marie's explanation for the home birth.

I asked about Liza, whether she would be present for the birth, and if so, who would be watching her. Marie said, "I'm almost certain that I want to be alone for this. I think I would be worrying too much about her if she were here. I need to do this thing myself." Her sister would take Liza when it was time.

We had gone into the bedroom, where the birth would take place. I gave them a list of equipment they would need and talked about what to expect. When Marie asked about positions in which to give birth, I demonstrated both squatting and kneeling, and explained that the choice would be hers, and that I would help her find the most comfortable way in which to deliver.

I examined Marie on her bed, with Alex and Liza watching intently. I listened to the sound of the fetal heartbeat, and then passed the stethoscope to Marie and Alex, and then to Liza.

Now, as I prepare for the birth, I run those memories through my mind. I leave the pool feeling calm, whole, reassured because I have not been paged. Taking my beeper from the front desk, I go home to call them.

At six in the evening I arrive at Marie and Alex's home, where I'm met also by Adrienne, the nurse who sometimes works with me. As I walk into the house and then into the bedroom, I feel the excitement of birth approaching. I feel the passion and spirit of life. Aware that I am about to be a part of a miracle, I feel privileged, but scared.

Marie is in the midst of a contraction when I come in. I say hello, and then turn to Adrienne to ask what is happening. Adrienne has just gotten there and has checked Marie's blood pressure. She has listened to the fetal heart rate and has done an internal exam. Marie's cervix is five centimeters dilated. Since by convention a fully dilated cervix is ten centimeters, Marie is halfway there.

Marie's contraction ends and she greets me with, "Glad you're here. I think this is the real thing." She is leaning back against the headboard of her bed, lovely and at ease, with hair in place, make-up on, wearing a pale-blue gown, and I am momentarily envious of a woman who can look so meticulously groomed while in labor.

"Adrienne tells me we may have a baby here tonight," I kid her. "You still feel like having another baby?"

"I think it's too late to change my mind, and anyway, the crib is set up, so I may as well go through with it." Alex is stretched out on the bed next to Marie. A contraction begins again. He puts his arm around her back and a hand on her abdomen, gently, and they both close their eyes and breathe slowly. When the contraction is over they open their eyes and join us again.

I go about setting out my equipment on the dresser near the bed. I have a head lamp, which I will plug into a wall outlet and wear so I can have light to work with. I take out the instruments to sterilize, the scissors, suction bulb, mucus trap, umbilical cord ties, cord clamps, and I put them aside. I set out a pile of sterile gloves and some oil for the perineal massage I will do as the baby's head stretches Marie's tissues.

Some of my setting up is just puttering. I put things out and chat with Marie and Alex between contractions. They are quite self-sufficient and seem to need little support from us. We try to be supportive but not intrusive.

I finish taking things out of my bag and go over to the bed to check Marie. I take her blood pressure. A contraction begins and I sit next to her with my hand resting on her abdomen. I feel the contraction and get a sense of what it is like. When it is over, I lean forward and listen with the stethoscope to the fetal heart.

I listen to the baby and think, we meet each other again. Sometimes I feel I know the baby well by the time it is born. I tell Marie and Alex, "It all seems fine," and then ask, "How are you feeling, Marie?"

A contraction is beginning and she can only nod to me as she closes her eyes and begins to breathe slowly, quietly, rhythmically. I get up gently from the bed and go to the kitchen where Adrienne joins me as I put the water on to boil. I'll use one pot to sterilize instruments. Another pot of water will be allowed to cool and then the water will be applied to Marie's perineum as the baby is being born. Marie's sister has come to take Liza. There is no one else in the house.

Adrienne and I make ourselves at home in the kitchen. We use the time to catch up on each other's lives. It can be lonely at a birth, without someone to consult, someone with whom to share worries and gain reassurances. Adrienne pours off some water to make tea. We talk about Marie and Alex and how well they are doing. We are both looking forward to the evening ahead.

We take our tea back up to the bedroom. Contractions have increased and Marie is becoming very uncomfortable. She cries out in pain. Alex holds her. I sit down on the bed next to her and take her hand. I tell her that she is okay, that she is doing beautifully, that it will soon be over. Adrienne brings a wet washcloth and wipes Marie's face. I look at Marie and I see the terror of childbirth in her eyes. I feel it. I remember it. I know it can be survived. I tell her that.

The contraction is at its peak. Marie's eyes meet mine and she is begging me to end it. I tell her again that she is okay, that I know how she feels, that she is doing magnificently.

The contraction ends and she rests. She rolls on her side to see if it will be better that way. The next contraction is on her already and she suddenly bolts back onto her back. For her it was worse on her side. She stiffens. Alex gives her their practiced signals of relaxation. She searches our faces for relief. Her body relaxes again. She rests.

Another contraction is upon her. This time she feels a sudden flood of liquid spilling out onto the bed. Her membranes have ruptured. The fluid is thin and clear and free of indicators of fetal difficulty. Three hours have passed since I arrived at the house. The birth will be soon. I replace the wet pads under her with dry ones. I listen again to the sound of the fetal heart. I am about to examine her internally to see how dilated her cervix has become, but a contraction begins and she yells out, "I have to push! I have to push!," and her face squeezes up and her eyes shut and a deep pushing grunt comes from somewhere deep inside of her. She is half sitting, propped up against the head-board of her bed and she is beginning to birth her baby. The contraction ends and this time she looks up and laughs. "Ooo, I couldn't help myself. I just had to push." I laugh with her and say, "I think it's getting close."

Adrienne brings the water from the kitchen. She soaks a pad in the water and then places the warm compress between Marie's legs. Marie finds the warmth soothing and asks for a fresh compress when this one cools. I put on my head lamp and get out the oils which I will use to massage her perineum as the baby is being born.

The contractions become less frequent but more intense. Marie complains, asks if anything is wrong. "Sometimes they just stretch out in the last few minutes," I tell her, "but at least that gives you a chance to rest a little more in between." Her contractions are now every four minutes instead of every two. Between them she rests, she talks with us, she adjusts her position, asks for a pillow to be shifted slightly. Night is coming and she is tired. As the world outside darkens and as the moments of birth approach, we focus our energy on Marie's laboring. A contraction comes; she grits her teeth and she pushes.

At first we see nothing except the straining of her muscles, then we see a bulging of the labia. On the next contraction there is a slight spreading apart of the labia, and on the next we see the fine hair of the baby. I dip my fingers in the oil and as the labia spread and the tissues stretch, I rub gently and strengthen the places that seem to be stretched to their limits. Between the contractions Adrienne continues to replace the warm compresses. She tells Marie, and Alex, who is beside her on the bed holding her, that their baby has fine dark hair.

Birth is a slow transition, a process. A contraction comes, Marie pushes, and we see the top of the baby's head; then she relaxes and the baby's head slides back into her. The next contraction, and her pushing and groaning that come with it, shows us more head than before, and after that contraction the baby's head slides back inside again, but not so far as it was before. The dome of head we see next gets larger and then retracts. The baby plays peek-a-boo with us and each time we wonder if that will be the moment of its birth.

Marie pushes and then lets go. She struggles with the work of birthing, caught in a will not totally hers. We tell her she can see the baby's head if she looks down during the contraction, but she shakes her head no. She is too much in it to observe. She pushes again, and then, on a signal from inside her, she lets go and the baby slides back inside her. I think of the baby saying, "No, not just yet. Give me another moment." I think of the mother wanting her baby, wanting to have it outside with her, also wanting still to hold it inside her body. She plays with it as it begins to be born. Are those her hugs the baby feels as it is pushed by the uterus and by the mother's pushing, hugs and squeezes along the way?

There is a moment when it happens by itself, a moment when the circle of head that comes through the vagina stretches the opening more and more. There is one moment when the mother screams, "It's coming!," when the head emerges, and then it is out too far to return. My hands, which have been massaging and supporting the tissues that were being stretched, now cradle the head as a wet and slippery baby slides gently out of its mother's body. We are all quiet. Marie looks down at her child lying on the bed between her legs. Alex leans over to see his son. Adrienne hands me a towel and I lift the baby who is now beginning to stir. He is beautiful. His skin is colors of pink and blue. His tiny fists are clenched. His face is serene, his eyes as yet unopened. His chest begins to move with the shallow breaths of a baby not yet unattached from the placenta and umbilical cord. I lift him in the towel and pass him to his mother, and as I do he takes his first deep breath and lets out a cry. His eyes open for a minute, his little arms extend outward and then come back against his chest. His cry, his surprise, are answered by his mother's arms, which take him, and she holds him close against her bare skin and he is soothed.

I look him over, at once a doctor looking at the physical signs of color and breathing pattern and muscle tone, and at the same time registering the wonderment of what I have just been a part of. Marie holds her baby. Alex places his pinky in his son's hand and lets the tiny fingers close over his.

The cord has stopped pulsating. I clamp and cut it, aware again that there is no turning back now. We must now commit ourselves to taking care of this child as well as his mother was able to do for the last nine months. That seems an awesome task. She has done so well.

Marie looks up at us and says, "He's so beautiful."

"Look at him looking at you," I add as the baby stares at his mother, then closes his eyes, and then searches again to meet her eyes.

Adrienne leans over and touches his fingers. "I think he looks like you, Marie."

"He's the spitting image of Liza when she was born," Marie tells us, examining the baby as she speaks.

I am sitting on the bed, soaked with the blood and amniotic fluid that came out with the baby. I warn Marie, "You are going to feel some cramps as the placenta separates from the uterus." We go on talking as she fondles the baby and we wait for the placenta to separate.

"Ow, it hurts," she tells me within minutes, and I see a trickle of blood and more of the umbilical cord being pushed out of her vagina, so I know the placenta has separated. I put my hand on her abdomen, and then use gentle traction on the cord to help the placenta come out.

"Ow, it hurts," she shrieks. "That hurts more than the baby."

Her tolerance for pain is gone. She has her baby now and this pain seems like an anticlimactic bother. It is out now, though. I examine it to be sure that all the parts are there, that the umbilical cord is normal, and then I look again to be sure that Marie is not bleeding.

It is ten o'clock. We are all quiet and reflective. There is now a new person here with us, but he does not seem like a stranger. It is as though someone we know has just come to join us.

Adrienne and I stay another hour at their home. After we wash the baby, Alex holds him while Adrienne takes Marie into the bathroom to help her shower. I gather the wet and bloody regular and plastic sheets together and remake the bed with fresh linens. I then examine the baby more thoroughly. I enjoy having a chance to hold him and talk to him. Alex watches the exam and then leaves me with the baby to go downstairs to bring up some food for Marie, who is suddenly very hungry.

Marie gets back into the clean bed and begins those awkward first attempts at nursing. Adrienne and I pack up our things and then we all just sit around talking for a while. Marie needs to talk about her labor, her fear, her thrill at being able to get through it all. "You know, Michelle, I was so scared because last time, when I had the anesthesia, I never felt the birth. I was afraid I wouldn't be able to do it. I wanted to feel strong but I wasn't sure I could."

"You did so well," we both tell her. I add, "It hurts. It hurts, but you can make it through."

"They don't really tell you that in the classes and the movies," Marie says. "They say, 'If you breathe right, it won't hurt,' and then when it hurts I feel something must be wrong or I'm not doing it right."

"Marie, the breathing and all the childbirth training are ways to help with the pain, but the pain is there and it is real."

"You know," she says, looking at each of us and then at her baby, "I felt like my body was being turned inside out."

Her baby is nursing now, quietly sucking and looking as though he had been doing this all his life. Alex is on the bed with them, his arm around his wife's shoulder. How peaceful they are, the three of them.

Adrienne and I go downstairs and sit out on the steps for a few minutes and talk with each other. We share both the pleasure and the relief that this birth went smoothly. Neighbors will be in to help Marie in the morning. Adrienne will visit in the evening, and I will be by on Tuesday to see how they are doing. They will call us if there are any questions or problems.

Adrienne and I say good night and give each other a hug to express the closeness we have in our work. Then we get in our cars and drive away.

I am tired, needing both solitude and sleep. I am glad it is nighttime, and that I do not have to be anywhere else right now. I want to be able to slowly separate myself from the evening, to replay what I want to, to work it over until it can all be put to rest and I am clear to go on.

It was a luxury I had in those days.

Chapter Six

I overslept this morning. When I woke up, it was light out. I had a feeling of panic because I couldn't remember what day it was or where I was or where I was supposed to be, but I knew something was wrong. I guess that is my system's reaction to what I am doing. I have to get myself together.

After two days on obstetrics, I have done three Caesarean sections and one vaginal delivery. Today I did two Caesareans with Neil Anderson, who explained that he tends to be aggressive with patient care. "And I don't give away any surgical material, since I want to maintain my skills," he told me over the operating table as we did the first section. "And I don't give anything away until I find out how conscientious a resident is."

I'm not sure that the second section was necessary. Anderson commented while we were doing it that he didn't quite believe the tracing on the monitor that seemed to indicate that the fetus was in distress. "May as well do it and get it over with, though," he added. Rarely do people listen with their ears. We act on the monitor, not on the patient. A woman is moved along like a machine, with her uterus split open, and almost no control over what is going on.

With the first section, the anesthesiologist failed to get the spinal needle in, so he told the woman he'd have to put her to sleep. The woman cried because that meant that her husband couldn't be there and because she wanted to be awake for the birth of her baby.

Fran has been at my house working steadily on the new health resources guides. Having raised her child, she now devotes all of her time to women's health issues. She is always working, and though it seems such a struggle to improve health care, she maintains both a cynicism and an optimism about what we can achieve. In spite of her reservations about my doing a residency, she repeatedly bolsters me up so I can go back for more. I think I am giving her another view of OB-GYN, which she knows mostly as an outsider. In the midst of our serious political-philosophical discussions, we sometimes run out shopping and enjoy discovering scouring pads for ten cents apiece or dresses for $8. Fran is from Everytown and knows every discount and bargain store in this area.

Today I called home and talked with Fran because I needed to share with someone outside what it is like for me here. I am so depressed over what I see happening: I no longer believe women can get proper care for labor and delivery in hospitals. I'm more confused than ever about where I am going. I have much less hope than before of surviving within the system.

I talked with Carol after Grand Rounds this morning and told her that I was feeling down and also confused about what my responsibilities were. She said I'm in charge of 3W and that Richard should have told me that. Even John is having trouble with Richard: he says that Richard doesn't want to know about patient problems, won't explain anything, and is totally centered on the paperwork of the service.

I just keep thinking about how hopeless it is, and how different I feel from when I began. I'm frightened by how far out of the system I feel. I wonder if I could practice in a hospital even if I got through training. It's not just my feminist perspective, but the whole realm of intuition, sensitivity and spirituality that has been destroyed in the medicalization of childbirth.

The process of birth and the continual emergence of one person out of the belly of another continues to overwhelm me and mystify me. It's a sacred act that has been turned into an

ugly ritual, not just because of the procedures—which are sometimes necessary and lifesaving—but because of the attitude
with which they are performed. It's like considering the beauty
of those moments when sexuality takes on a spiritual quality and
comparing that with fucking, with pornography. The medical
birth is pornographic. The woman is degraded. The physician
intimidates her and forcefully takes from her both the act of
birth and that which she herself has nurtured. All day long I
watch women who have been violated and who don't even
know it.

I long for my patients in New Jersey, and for my children of
home birth. I wonder if we can create new institutions. I wonder if I'll be destroyed in the process.

The whole experience today was like taking part in some
great sacrificial ritual in which women come forth and sacrifice
themselves and their newborns.

Thursday   *Day 46*

I've gotten myself together enough to do my work. Richard's
lack of supervision has its advantages because I am freer to do
what I think I should. I feel comfortable doing postpartum care.
I am learning a great deal about fevers and postpartum complications.

My score is now four sections and one vaginal delivery. Today
I scrubbed with Larry Morris, who explained that he would be
doing the procedure and that I would get to do little of it. When
it was over he said, "I had not realized how proficient you are.
From now on I'll let *you* do them." I don't feel that proficient,
but what I do feel is a closeness with what I am doing.

Friday morning   *Day 47*

I thought I was okay yesterday, but I wasn't. I went home and
thought of all the things I had to do, but I just collapsed. I was
distressed that there weren't any groceries in the house, and I
felt burdened by the whole household. I knew I was unreason-

able, and went to bed. I got up for supper and went back to bed, and then got up about an hour later when Maggie's barking woke me. By then I was feeling better, but I was bothered because I knew I was reacting to the day, and that I had just kept everything inside.

When I tried to sleep I kept thinking about the section I had done with Larry. After the baby had been delivered, I reached in to remove the placenta and to explore the interior of the uterus. I felt a thinned-out portion at the top of the uterus. The woman had had an abortion ten years ago in Puerto Rico. They operated through her abdomen and apparently cut across the top of her uterus in order to remove the fetus. This woman might not have survived a vaginal delivery. My shock was overwhelming because I am afraid that illegal, inept abortions will become common again if women lose control over their reproductive rights and if the "right-to-lifers" win on the abortion issue. As a physician, I see their position as demanding the "right to death," which this botched-up woman almost suffered.

Later

When I saw Carol on L&D at noontime, I started to cry. She took me into the supply closet and I wept for a long time, flooded with experience and emotion.

I had two difficult deliveries with Richard. He stops me from doing what I am used to doing, and then I lose my rhythm and I feel thrown off. It's like driving a car one way for ten years, and then, as you are approaching an intersection and trying to brake the car, having someone say, "No, use the other foot to stop it." Richard is so invested in how he wants something done, he forgets there is a baby there. One of the babies needed to be suctioned and I had to remind him to do it.

"Catching a baby is like catching a football" was what we were taught in medical school. "You catch it and hold it in the crook of your arm and close to your body." The one-armed baby catch is designed for hospitals where the woman is up in the air and the doctor needs one hand free to cut the cord, suction, etc. I used to be good at it, but over the last few years, delivering babies at home, I have become accustomed to using two hands. I had become accustomed to babies coming out onto a bed or on sheets on a floor, with a rhythm more peaceful than exists in a delivery room.

It's the episiotomy, though, that bothers me so much, and since my difficulty with Hilda the first day, Richard and the others are watching to be sure that I will do them. I can't get used to them, though. The women spend three, four, five miserable days postpartum with the episiotomy pain being the most difficult part of it all. Their hemorrhoids are bad, their episiotomies are swollen, and they have difficulty walking and sitting.

Since the episode with Hilda Cameron on Tuesday when she had to take the scissors from my hand, I felt I had two choices, because everyone quickly knew what had happened: I could either let people think I was incompetent—that after ten years of delivering babies I didn't know how to do an episiotomy— or tell them what I think and have some of them write me off as crazy.

A nurse asked about "pelvic relaxation," a loosening of the musculature of the vaginal area which has been attributed to not having an episiotomy. I told her that 1) it has never been proven that the two are related; 2) I was concerned about the degree to which women were debilitated postpartum because of the episiotomy; 3) women spend a major portion of their pregnancy worried about whether they will have one and what it will feel like; 4) women are never given a choice in the matter —it is the doctor who decides. The doctor says, "I'll only do it if I have to," and the woman feels reassured—except that episiotomy is done 99 percent of the time and few doctors seem to know how to deliver a baby without doing one.

I want those obstetricians to stop cutting open women's vaginas. Childbirth is not a surgical procedure. This time in the hospital has made that far more clear to me than it ever was before.

It's been years since I've cried as much as I have in the last week. I really don't know if I can go through with it.

I recouped a little over the weekend. I talked yesterday on the phone with Martha, a lay midwife with whom I worked in New Jersey. She said, "Hang in there, Michelle, and learn what you can. We're all waiting for you." I need to keep my sense of purpose in what I am doing. I have to do episiotomies. I have to play the game better than I have been doing.

Martha herself is in need of support. She is practicing illegally and is terrified about the outcome of a case in California, where a midwife is being tried for murder. The baby she helped deliver was doing poorly at birth but was resuscitated by the midwife and then transferred by ambulance to the hospital. It died several days later. It is not clear when the baby became worse, or why. The pressure against home birth is increasing, though.

I have hit every red light on the way to work this morning, which has never happened before. I think I'm going to be late. Because it is Sunday, I'll be the only resident on OB, with Flo covering as chief for the day.

On the way home

It was an easy day at work, with only one delivery early in the morning. I was called suddenly to the delivery room while still making rounds, and I arrived in time to watch a midwife deliver a baby. The woman had been rushed back to the delivery room because the fetal monitor had shown some patterns of distress, but the baby was fine at birth. The midwife had made a large episiotomy because she wanted to get the baby out quickly, but it didn't bother me. It was needed. After the delivery the midwife turned to me and asked, "Do you want to sew up the episiotomy?" I didn't know if I was being dumped on or given an honor. I sewed it up, though, and the attending, Dr. Curry, approved of my work.

● ● ●

That afternoon I did an oxytocin challenge test (OCT)—performed by the nurses during the week but by the residents on weekends. It is a test of how the fetus is doing in utero. We give the woman enough of the drug pitocin intravenously to cause her uterus to contract. Then we put a monitor on her abdomen to record the fetal heart rate and to see if the pitocin is causing a pattern suggestive of fetal distress. If the test is positive—that is, if there is distress—then the woman will be delivered in the next day or so. If it is negative, she is allowed to go on with the pregnancy. Flo was an unexpectedly good teacher. She tends to do things "by the book," but that is exactly what I am here to learn. Sometimes she is like a walking textbook as she lists off protocols of how to manage obstetrical problems. Short, slight, somewhat remote and aloof, she does not seem to mix with the other residents. She was quite friendly with me, though, making the day better than many others.

I also "labor-sat" today with a patient who was getting pitocin in order to induce labor. That is a procedure usually done during the week too, when there is enough staff around. If a woman is getting pitocin, a physician has to be on the L&D suite because of the dangers of the drug. If the doctor has to go to the floors to take care of other patients, then the pitocin must be turned off. A nurse must be in the room at all times too, as long as the pitocin is being given through the IV.

At four o'clock the nurse who came on duty refused to carry out the pitocin order as it was written, which was the way the attending (who is very intervention-oriented) had told me to write it. Margaret, the nurse, said, "If that's the way you want it written, that's fine, but I'm not giving it in that dose." I told her that I respected her decision and in fact agreed it was too much, but that I had to write the order.

"Why don't you just write it as you were instructed to and then not pay attention to what I do about it?" was her suggestion.

"Sure," I told her, "and I won't even ask any questions about how much is already in the bottle."

The patient had been on pitocin all day and had earlier shown signs of difficulty with the drug, so it had been stopped and then restarted. "I'm going off duty now," I told her, "but you're in good hands here. You have a nurse who cares."

Pitocin, a colorless drug, is widely used to induce labor and to speed it along. It can also cause fetal distress and rupture of the uterus. A professor of obstetrics at the medical school once said, "If they were to put a dye in the pitocin, you'd see it in the IV of almost every woman in the country who is in labor."

Monday morning   *Day 50*

I drove home after work last night to pick up Heather to take her with me to a pot-luck supper at Carol's, but then didn't really feel like going out. Gail, Arlene and I moved bookcases and unpacked the stereo and set it up in the living room. It seemed so lovely and friendly and cozy and warm at home. Gail has fit into the household so well and Arlene is working out wonderfully as a baby-sitter.

The party was a stiff, uncomfortable event, for which few people showed up. I stayed up late talking with Carol. Heather curled up in my lap, I took out my knitting, and Carol worked on the afghan she was making. It was quiet and peaceful, almost like being at home.

I feel bad about Carol. For one thing, she is very isolated. She lives with other people, trying to carry the same domestic load as they do and keep up her end of the housework, but they do not understand the strains on her due to her work or her fatigue. She once told me about bursting into tears in the grocery store because she had been awake for two nights straight and suddenly couldn't cope with the line for weighing vegetables.

Carol is isolated at work too, not yet having found where she fits in. I think it will happen, though, especially if she can create an out-of-hospital birth center when she finishes next year. I'm envious of how far along she is.

On the way home

I had several patients in labor at the same time today. One woman, a patient of Dr. Carter's, wanted no anesthesia, no episiotomy, no IVs, etc. She was there with her husband and a woman who had come as a labor coach. We were all hoping she would deliver precipitously in bed before her doctor could get there and take her back to the delivery room, but Ian Dorsi, who was covering for Carter, arrived.

The delivery started out fine. We were all back in the delivery room, the patient up in stirrups, and Dorsi and I were both at her perineum. I was feeling on top of what I was doing and proud that I knew what I knew. This woman wanted the kind of delivery I was more accustomed to. The head was coming out and I was commenting under my breath that the woman had plenty of room and that her tissue was thinning out fine. I was hoping Dorsi wouldn't do an episiotomy, since she didn't want one. Dorsi muttered angrily to me, "This isn't my first delivery, you know!" After the head came out, he turned it to the left and then told me to do the same. When I tried to turn the head further, it wouldn't go and he got mad and said I was turning it the wrong way, which was the way he showed me to. It's really hard when someone interferes in the middle of the delivery, because I was trying to follow what he was telling me to do. The atmosphere was pretty strained after that.

There is no clarity as to who delivers the baby. I've been told that the residents deliver the babies, but the attendings are there, and rightfully so, to deliver their own patients. I am part of a huge fraud.

I had a good delivery later on with Dr. Core. I had gotten worried about the monitor pattern, which showed severe slowing of the fetal heart rate. I tried to get Richard to look at it and tell me what was going on, but he wouldn't answer my questions. He just told me not to worry. I ended up going back into the delivery room with Dr. Core, which I was especially anxious to do, since she was thinking of putting on forceps to get the baby out. She used local anesthesia and did a large episiotomy and was helpful in showing me how she does the repair. We had a nice talk about obstetrics and men, and I told her I was doing a part-time residency. She's an interesting woman who did her training later in life. She spent many years in Africa doing hundreds of deliveries and she has a different perspective on obstetrics.

Tuesday   *Day 51*

Heather lost her first tooth, and she also really lost it! Late last night we made a picture of the tooth and left it with a note for the tooth fairy. This morning at five when I went in to put the money under her pillow, I was unable to find the note. I left the money, anyway.

On the way home

I'm becoming overtly irritated with Richard's reluctance to teach. I'm going to tell him that he's got to explain things to me if I'm going to manage patients, otherwise I'm just doing his scut work. Today I took a delivery back without him and he was really pissed afterward. The woman was having her eighth baby and I knew she was going to be okay. It was a nice delivery and there were no problems. I was just glad to be there.

I did a delivery with Dr. Jackson, who, instead of scrubbing, just watched while I delivered. I did an episiotomy as I was supposed to and then sewed it up.

I think that the acute crisis is over and that I will be doing all right with obstetrics.

Dr. Pierce announced yesterday that there will be another part-time resident, Karen Dole, joining the program in two weeks. I met her last week when she came for an interview. I guess I have mixed feelings about her. I think her arrival will take some of the heat off me because with both of us working two-thirds time, there will be more help than if there were one full-time person instead of us. I also worry, though, that she is one more person "like them" who will thus make me feel even more isolated.

There is a way in which physicians are made to resemble one another. Learning to act like a doctor is a less obvious part of the long educational process, and one which seems to happen spontaneously. Although I have been deeply committed to the work of medicine, I have never been a product of that mold which makes all doctors seem the "same" rather than "other," and which would cause other physicians to think of me as the "same" rather than "other."

Karen is friendly and assertive, with an air of self-confidence. She is coming from a full-time position in another residency so she can work part-time. She has three young children and a husband, and a baby-sitter who has been part of her family for years.

I'm hoping that Karen's arrival will allow me to cut back to the two-thirds time I am supposed to be working. I would like to stay home on Sundays, at least for part of the day. I would still come in at six, but then I could leave when she arrives.

I spent time with a fourteen-year-old who was in labor. She was in the hospital with her father, having a baby which she wanted to give up for adoption but which her father wanted to keep and raise. He came out of her room and talked with me for a few minutes while the nurses were busy with her; otherwise he stayed with his daughter. She wanted to be asleep for the delivery because she didn't want to see the baby. The anesthesiologist said she could only have general anesthesia if she had nothing else for pain. This is, actually, safe medical practice, but I have seen physicians, time and time again, give pain medication to a woman who will be having general anesthesia.

Every time this frightened girl screamed out with pain, she was offered the choice of relief then or being asleep for the delivery. I think they were just punishing her. When she was almost fully dilated she finally broke down and begged for relief. They gave her an epidural, which stopped her labor. As I left for the day, they were getting ready to do a section on her. I was furious because she was so close to making it through. They will do the section with the epidural anesthesia and she will be awake and will have to see and/or hear the baby at birth.

Wednesday, on the way home   *Day 52*

I like being alone on L&D, as I was Sunday, more than when Richard is around and harassing me, as he was today. I have a patient on 3W who has an abscess, and Richard claims she does not. We got a culture back showing infectious organisms, but Richard is still refusing to accept that she has an infection.

I took care of a patient with elevated blood pressure, and two with prolonged ruptured membranes. Usually the membranes around the baby and the fluid rupture shortly before or during labor. Once they have ruptured there is a somewhat higher possibility of infection, made even higher by vaginal exams. The definition of "prolonged" has changed over the past fifteen years from 72 hours being considered "prolonged" when I was in medical school to 48 hours when I practiced in South Carolina, to 12–24 hours at present. Once doctors define the woman as having prolonged ruptured membranes, the delivery of the baby is begun, either by induction of labor with pitocin or Caesarean section.

There is a contradiction which everyone seems to ignore regarding how often one does vaginal examinations during labor. Although the exams are a source of infection for both mother and baby, residents are required to examine women frequently in order to "chart" the progression of labor. I didn't do a lot of vaginal exams today and sometimes it was only toward the end that we discovered that a woman was in late stages of labor or near delivery time.

At Doctors Hospital we use Hill's chart of labor, a curve developed by Dr. Ernest Hill which defines on a graph how a labor should progress. Each woman's chart has a blank graph of hours and of centimeters of cervical dilation which we must record approximately hourly in order to evaluate the shape of her labor curve. When a woman's labor is off the "proper" curve, she is subjected to intervention in several possible forms.

Dr. Irv Warren did an interesting delivery with me watching. We were at the perineum and he was seated. I was standing as close as I could, trying to move away some of the things he'd put between me and the patient. He suddenly turned to me and said, "Would you do an episiotomy?" I felt that as a very loaded question, but answered, "All I can do is speak from my own experience, which has been not to do episiotomies for the past few years." I felt set-up, and I didn't know what was coming.

Warren went on, "What would you do instead of an episiotomy?"

"I'd do perineal massage."

He asked what I meant and wanted me to show him. I told him it was a technique I'd learned from the midwives. He said, "Well, do it."

I felt bad for the woman and her husband. They were aware of something going on, although they couldn't quite catch what was being said. I told Dr. Warren that I didn't feel comfortable doing perineal massage in this situation. I added, "I've never done it with a woman up in stirrups."

"What position were they in? Left lateral?" He was referring to a woman being on her side when she delivers.

"No, I have done it that way, but mostly they were squatting or kneeling on their knees."

"But where were you then?"

"Underneath," I answered.

Warren did the episiotomy. He did the delivery. As the woman was pushing he suddenly started to yell at her to push harder. I was angry and wanted to ask what made him feel he had the right to shout.

After the delivery Warren said, "You'll have your chance another time," referring to my showing him perineal massage. I said, "Maybe in the Alternative Birth Service one day."

While Warren's patient was in labor, the monitor had been recording a slowing of the fetal heart rate from 140/min. to 60/min. Apparently as long as the rate picks up again quickly this is not considered a problem. I wish I'd known that during my time at home births when I would become alarmed at any drop. I'm learning so much more now. It's not that I would take more chances, but I would develop a better system of knowing what is going on.

I like working with this department's criteria of labor and of good and poor progress. It is a system that assists in defining what is going on and what actions should or should not be taken. This is what I wanted to be learning when I came here.

Later in the day I talked with Carol about Warren's delivery. She told me to be careful of him. "His pattern is to be very friendly," she said, "and then to start screaming, and then to feel guilty and apologize for how he acted but to say he had to act that way." I remember now that he once did that with Barbara in the OR and I heard her telling him that she didn't think he should be yelling at her. I wonder if he'll yell at me. Sometimes my age is an advantage.

Heather misses me a lot on school holidays like today. Christmas and Easter will be difficult for her this year, but by next year I hope to be able to get vacation time.

Thursday   *Day 53*

I realized last evening that my house in New Jersey was supposed to have been sold by now. I didn't get a call from my mother, so I don't know what's going on and I'm afraid to find out. If it's bad news, I don't feel like coping with it. I feel overwhelmed by financial pressures because I don't have the money to do this for more than one year. After that I'll probably have to moonlight.

Last evening I dropped off the fireplace damper at a welder's and then went on to say hello to Laurie. I enjoyed being out in the evening alone casually visiting without Heather. Laurie gave me some papers about the midwife trial in California. The baby was born with a true knot in the cord. As the baby was being born, the knot tightened and stopped the blood supply. The baby died in the hospital six days later.

Last week we did a Caesarean, and that baby also had a true knot in the cord, but the section was being done for other reasons. When we delivered the baby out of the woman's abdomen the attending saw the knot and said, "This baby wouldn't have made it vaginally." If that baby had died in the hospital during a vaginal delivery, no one would have been tried for murder. In fact, even negligence in hospitals is rarely questioned and is often covered up.

Heather fussed at me a lot last night and was very cranky. It seems to me that happens on days when she is home and I am working, as on school holidays. She keeps asking about my being so busy and last night in bed asked, "Are you going to be this busy next summer?" I told her I didn't know, but the truth is that I will be, and I feel terrible about it. I am going to have to provide her with as much support as I can from others, to make up for my own absence.

Later

The day began with a direct confrontation with Richard about the, for him, nonexistent abscess. When I arrived on the floor at six this morning the nurse reported that the abscess had burst and had drained a large amount of pus. Richard and I looked at the abscess site, and he claimed again that it was not an abscess. I told him, "You can call it what you like, but where I come from, when pus comes out of a pocket and it's the only positive culture we get from the lab, then it's an abscess."

I was so discouraged that I took my time making rounds on the rest of the patients, but since I had to be on L&D by eight, I had to finish seeing them later in the day.

I scrubbed this morning on a section with Dr. Joseph, and discovered after we were in the operating room that he was letting me do the surgery. The woman had spinal anesthesia and was awake so I couldn't tell Dr. Joseph this was my first time doing a section. When I told him later he was surprised and said he had seen worse from people much further along.

Later in the day I examined a patient and told Richard that her cervix was eight to nine centimeters dilated. He then examined her and said that I was wrong, that she was only six centimeters and at −1 to −2 station, meaning that the head was still high up in the pelvis. I had said she was at 0 to +1, which is much farther down. Dr. Dorsi, worried about the lack of progress of his patient if Richard was correct, went in to check her himself. "Richard," he said, "she's nine centimeters, and in fact she's almost fully dilated. Have you forgotten how to examine a woman?" He was teasing Richard, and I took the opportunity to join in. I think if I just give Richard enough room, he will do himself in. It's not that it's so hard to be wrong, but Richard is very sharp and it's his determination to prove me wrong that is so irritating.

I think I am surviving here by tuning out certain people, including my worry about the way patients are treated. I'm keeping the distance I need in order to get through. I concentrate a lot on what I want to do in the future. I have to go on learning because I want to share what I know. There is so much more I'll be able to do for women's health if I can get this training.

Friday   *Day 54*

Last night I drove out to a wallpaper store with Heather and finally picked out paper. I got a burlap-type grasscloth, which will be a wonderful soft background for pictures and posters in the dining room. I'm planning to put it up this weekend. It feels good to have resolved that conflict.

I found myself last night thinking about the day and the

Caesarean I had done. Performing a Caesarean is the one time that truly gives you the feeling of delivering the baby. I remember having my hand in the uterus. Pressure was being applied by Dr. Joseph at the top of the uterus while my hand grasped the head of the baby and assisted it out through the incision. I felt a sense of excitement and of power and of personal accomplishment that is not present in a vaginal birth. This is the time the *obstetrician* truly delivers the baby; in a vaginal birth, it is the mother.

These feelings of mine help me in trying to understand current obstetrical practices, and the spiraling increase in Caesareans. I have a vivid recollection of cutting through the uterus and first seeing the membranes bulging. I was so proud of myself for the fine surgery involved in cutting so delicately so as not to rupture the membranes yet.

I watched two deliveries today. One of the babies was born with a lot of meconium, and I was surprised that no attempt was made to suction the baby before it took its first breath. The meconium is the baby's first stool, and sometimes it is passed while the baby is in utero. A baby who breathes it into its lungs can die from the pneumonia-type reaction that is produced. The delivery table didn't even have the suction trap out. Later I talked with Art, one of the other residents, who has had a lot of training in pediatrics, and he agreed that the baby should have been suctioned immediately. He recounted to me his numerous unsuccessful attempts to get the OB department to stock the suction traps. When I delivered babies at home I always had one suction set open, ready to use if I needed it. I think that in the hospital they don't worry as much because they think that if the baby gets sick, then they'll just treat it.

This morning I made rounds on twenty-five patients in two hours. It's a testimony only to the poor care we give.

Adrienne came for the weekend. We went to the ballet Saturday evening, and yesterday Adrienne came to work with me for a few hours. Her presence made it harder for me to slide into the routine, to shut my eyes to what I am now a part of.

I can intellectually explain why I am doing this, why I have to learn to use the fetal monitors, but I don't feel right inside. Adrienne is trying to get into midwifery school, in which case she will face many of the same issues. What she and I were able to do at home births is not taught in any school and is discouraged in almost all of them.

Adrienne and I have talked of someday practicing together again. She would be a midwife; I, as an obstetrician, would take care of her high-risk patients, the ones for whom a home birth is not safe. I want to be that person in the hospital who can carry on the work and caring of midwives who deliver women at home.

I don't like being at work Sundays. I feel deprived of the rest of my life. Yet I was torn leaving the hospital yesterday because there was a woman in labor with twins, both of whom were in a breech position, and another woman having her first baby, also in a breech position. Both women will probably be sectioned. I didn't want to leave, but once I was on my way home, I was glad to be gone.

I have learned that some of the other residents do not see the twenty-five patients they are supposed to see in the morning. Art told me he could make rounds in twelve minutes just by walking down the hall and shaking hands with patients. I had thought, however, that Beth, another of the residents, was very conscientious, since her notes were always comprehensive. On one patient yesterday I read the note Beth wrote Saturday morning, which said: "Perineum fine." I turned to the patient and said, "Did the doctor check your episiotomy yesterday?" The patient looked at me and said, "Oh no, nobody's checked me since my delivery." I guess Beth isn't checking everyone. I'm not checking every patient either. I can't in the two hours I have.

Checking twenty-five women correctly would take three to four hours. It takes a long time just for a woman to turn over or to take off her underpants or pad for me to see the episiotomy. The pain keeps her from being able to move quickly. Sometimes the babies are in the bed with the mothers, either being held or nursed, and then it takes even longer to move the woman into position to be checked.

It can take half an hour to properly take care of one woman with post-Caesarean infection or other complications. In addition to locating the source of the problem, cultures must be taken, blood tests ordered or done, and questions answered.

Yesterday I had a long talk with Jessica, the fourteen-year-old who had a section last week. She talked about what it was like to have her family want to keep the baby, while she herself would rather forget it all and go back to her life in Utah. I supported the reality of her difficult position, and I used what has become my standard approach to an unwanted pregnancy. An unwanted pregnancy has no good solution. Whatever the choice, the price is high: for abortion, for having a child and giving it up, or for trying to raise a child that is not wanted.

This girl's situation is made sadder by the degree to which the family wants her to keep the baby. I happened to walk by the nursery while Jessica and her father were there. The grandfather was crying. We were all talking about how cute the baby was, and I agreed that the little girl did look like the grandfather.

Later in the day, when I talked with Jessica, I told her that it was important for the baby, at some point, to get to a home of her own. If Jessica wasn't going to keep her, she needed to make a decision. She asked me when I thought she should decide. The advice I gave her was: after three to four months. I know that social agencies usually say six months; they feel that by six months a baby has established a personal relationship with his or her caretakers. I know that the relationship happens

127

sooner, but I was trying to measure between this young girl's needs, what I thought was best for the baby, and what the agencies would be telling her.

Tonight I'm going to a dinner of the Obstetrical Society, and I'm sorry I agreed to go. I would rather be home.

On the way home

I was summoned quickly back to L&D from 3W because the nurse couldn't hear a fetal heart with a stethoscope. I thought of the possibilities: the fetal heart might be fine, but the nurse might not be picking it up with whatever instrument she was using to listen. The other possibility was that the baby was in trouble in utero. The most likely cause of that would be a prolapsed cord, where the cord comes through the cervix before the baby, and then when the baby's head comes down it presses on the cord and shuts off the blood supply to the baby. The rule is: "Once you feel the cord, you keep your hand in the vagina and try to hold the head up, away from the cervix, and the cord from being compressed by the head." The woman's bed will be tilted so she is head downward, and then gravity helps relieve the pressure of the baby's head on the cord. The woman is then taken immediately to the OR for the Caesarean, with someone's hand in the vagina. Even while she is prepped and draped, there is a nurse or doctor under the sheets holding the baby's head up until the baby is taken out by section.

I dashed into the room and did a pelvic exam, but I didn't feel a prolapsed cord. As it turned out, the baby was all right.

I had a discussion with Harriet, one of the midwives, about positions for childbirth. When I told her I had done home births for a couple of years, she muttered under her breath that she wished she could go to one. That had been Carol's response too. I have an experience behind me which others are frightened to have but are also envious of.

Harriet would like to be able to have siblings present at births in the Alternative Birth Service. I told her about the workshop

I had last year for children who had attended births. I wanted Heather and other children like her to have the chance to talk together about a common experience they could not easily talk about elsewhere. Harriet is hoping that when they get another midwife at the hospital they can do a research project on children being present for childbirth, which is the only way she can manage having children present.

Today I was supposed to be in Los Angeles speaking on "Feminism and Childbirth" at the American Public Health Association meeting. I had made that commitment before I took this position. Fran will be there and will speak for me.

My ability to take this program has necessitated a distancing from patients. I think about them, and care about them sometimes, but not the way I used to. I rarely know the names of the women I deliver. I do not see myself as an individual, nor can I be responsible for what I am doing. I see myself filling a certain role, without a name, without being anybody. Sometimes I am ashamed of myself as I walk into a room and realize I may have delivered the baby of the woman in that room.

Often I don't like the women I've delivered. I don't like them for their submissiveness. When I make rounds in the morning I ask, "When are you going home?" They answer, "I don't know when my doctor will let me."

They have let themselves be imprisoned. For me, the submissiveness of one woman becomes my own, as though we were all one organism. Their imprisonment adds to my own sense of powerlessness in this hospital. In my childhood, I had a tough bravado. I was forever the defender of the underdog, the kid who was being picked on. My mother would say, "You'll fight the battle of anyone who'll hold your jacket for you." When I was nine and lived in the city, I belonged to a "street gang." Having been told that red ants bite people, we spent many afternoons searching pavement and bushes for red ants we could destroy before they could hurt anyone.

In this environment, though, I am often depleted and then I can help neither myself nor anyone else. I do understand these women, but I don't want them to be weak. I want them to be strong for themselves and for me.

Tuesday, on the way home   *Day 58*

Barbara took me aside this morning and said everyone was aware of how unfair Richard is being to me. I was scheduled to scrub on a section with Jackson, who lets residents do a lot. Then at the last minute Richard sent me in with Dr. Black instead, and let John go with Jackson. As it turned out, Black, who is not known for letting residents do much, let me operate a lot, including opening and closing the uterus. Richard was surprised later when I told him what a good experience I'd had with Black.

I was sent next to the teen-age pregnancy clinic, where I enjoyed having time to spend with patients. I was doing the same thing I have done for years, but this time I had a specialist to ask when I had questions.

Thursday   *Day 60*

After work yesterday I stopped at the Sears surplus store and picked up a fireplace screen and andirons. Last night we burned newspaper and a part of a log. I've never had a fireplace before. The night before last I picked up the newly welded fireplace damper, and then crawled up under the chimney and installed it myself.

Today I watched Dr. Ingle put on forceps. He called the woman "sweetie," "honey" and "dearie." She was so thankful to him and told him to do anything he had to. The baby's head was already visible and the woman was pushing well. Then Dr. Ingle called for an extra dose of the epidural anesthesia to decrease her pain and make it easier to do an episiotomy. As the drug became effective, the woman's pushing became ineffective. She still tried to push but there was no longer any motion of her muscles. Dr. Ingle said, "Dearie, we may have to take the baby if you can't push any better." The woman tried but it was clear she was getting nowhere.

Dr. Ingle took the forceps, large stainless-steel instruments that, when hooked together, look like those plastic salad tongs with scissor handles. The baby's head fits between the two tongs. Then he took the handles in his hands, and using his full body weight, pulled the baby's head out. It took force, although everyone says you don't really have to pull hard. But his leg was braced on the table to give himself extra leverage as he leaned back and pulled. The muscles of his face were squeezed tight, sweat dripped from his forehead, and the baby was dragged out from the grateful mother. She had been pushing so beautifully before they gave her that extra dose.

I will have to learn to put on forceps. I can't imagine ever pulling on a baby's head that hard, but I guess I'll learn that too.

I went to a high-risk clinic and saw a sixteen-year-old with heart disease. We couldn't figure out how someone could be seven months pregnant and not have had the heart problem followed. We were about to order tests when we discovered that her heart disease is being carefully followed at another hospital, only we didn't have the records. That seems to happen all the time, as patients, especially poor patients, are sifted through the system of hospitals and clinics in the city.

I discharged a postpartum patient who had been anxious and seemingly worried about taking care of her baby. She had apparently been visited a few hours after she had delivered, by a woman in a white coat, who introduced herself as a doctor and said, "You've had four abortions. You're single. Are you sure you want to keep this baby, or do you want to give it up?" The patient had been afraid for these past three days that the baby would be taken away from her. The roommate had heard the whole exchange and finally told the nurses about it just before the patient was leaving. I talked with the roommate and with the nurses. We thought at first it was someone who didn't belong on the floor or in the hospital but had managed to see the chart. From the description of the woman, though, it was probably one of the attending doctors who has very strong beliefs about marriage and children. It seems worse that it was not an impostor.

Friday

I arrived home last night to discover that Heather had a badly inflamed eye. I began applying antibiotic ointment, and then, last night, I heard her screaming in her sleep. I went into her room to bring her to my bed and she was screaming, "No!" ... "Don't" ... "Stop it!" When I woke her at five this morning to put in more medicine she began screaming in the same way, so I guess that's what was frightening her. I held her until she fell back to sleep, and then left.

Yesterday Murray Avery gave a conference on fetal monitoring where he discussed the presumed mechanisms of control of fetal heart rate. I suddenly realized that these doctors are not obstetricians—i.e., people who take care of pregnant women— but pre-birth pediatricians, or what I call "feteotricians." The doctors have set up a relationship between themselves and the unborn child that does not include the mother. If these doctors don't care whether a woman uses natural childbirth or has epidural anesthesia, it is only because she has been written off, and her experience, whether she is awake or asleep, is irrelevant. She is the maternal environment. They are frustrated only that they cannot control her more.

On the way home

I had two deliveries today. The first was a woman who came in fully dilated and delivered quickly. I did an episiotomy, as I was supposed to. It was her third child and she didn't need it.

The second was a woman who came in almost fully dilated. Dr. Jackson ruptured her membranes and then put on the internal monitor, since there was some meconium staining of the fluid. I put a suction tube on the table and he suctioned the baby as soon as its head was out. The baby's shoulders tore through the episiotomy and then extended through her rectum. Now I have been taught to sew those tears. I never had a tear like that before I came here. It never happened in South Carolina and it never happened at home births. In those situations, the woman did not tear because I, as her physician, was more attuned to the natural pace of the birth. No one was shouting at her to "push harder" before the tissue had been slowly stretched by the baby's head or supported by my massage.

Saturday   *Day 62*

I took Heather to see *The Sound of Music* last night. Parenthood is difficult when one suddenly has to explain wars and killing. Heather is full of questions and ready to learn about the rest of the world, and I am reluctant to tell her. She has been sheltered by our lack of TV. She is a gentle child who doesn't hit others, who will give a toy to a friend who wants it, and who seems oblivious to violence.

On the way home

I was feeling high this morning when I went to L&D at eight. I had finished rounds early on 3W and then had gone on to help out on 3E where we keep patients when we are overcrowded.

Barbara, who was going off duty after the night, called me aside to talk. "Michelle, I think you should work late next Sunday," she said. Barbara is a friendly woman with soft features, but only coldness and anger showed on her face this morning.

"I thought we settled that weeks ago. I can't work those hours. I need to be home. What's happening next week?"

"Nothing, except Beth is tired of working those hours and she is becoming very resentful of you." Barbara and Beth have been working together at night. I imagined long hours of their complaining about my hours.

"When I took this job two months ago, the agreement was that I wouldn't work evenings on OB. I come in six mornings a week at six, but I go home at five. Beth agreed to cover those hours and she'll be getting that time back when Karen starts."

The high I had felt from my early-morning accomplishment was gone. I had finished my work and had gone on to help the others, but I still wasn't doing enough. I felt defeated. I had deluded myself into believing I could be accepted by the others, even with my limitations.

"I can't do it," I started to say, and then the weight of the past few weeks came tumbling down on me and I cried in defeat. Barbara sat down beside me and I tried to tell her what it was like for me. "I feel spread so thin. Arlene, my baby-sitter, told me last night she won't work any more weekends." I told her that Arlene had been staying out at night and just barely making it back by the time I left at a quarter of six. I needed to do something about a baby-sitter.

"Barbara, do you know what it's like getting up at five and waking Heather to put medicine in her eye and listening to her cry and having to go off to work? There just isn't any more of me to go around. Of course I'd like to help Beth. Of course I don't want the others to resent me. I can't do any more, though."

"I know that. I'm sorry. It's just that I'm on with Beth at night and I see how she resents those extra three hours on Sunday, and I just thought you could offer to work for her. I've offered to work but Richard won't let me. He won't let anyone else cover and he's making Beth take the full brunt of your being part-time. He won't even let me make rounds for you when you go to Chapel Hill, and I make rounds other times."

I was to give a talk, "Childbirth: In and Out of Hospitals," at the School of Public Health in Chapel Hill, North Carolina, a commitment made before I came to Doctors Hospital, and one which Dr. Pierce had assured me I could still keep. Richard was making my day's absence an issue, although he couldn't stop me from being away.

"There's nothing I can do about Beth or Richard. I'm working as much as I can." I told Barbara how I had tried unsuccessfully to get Carol to give Beth a whole day off in exchange for those hours.

A lingering sense of defeat stayed with me the rest of the day.

I admitted a woman for evaluation of her high blood pressure and could not hear the fetal heart at all. I took her to L&D, and when I left they had still not been able to hear the heart even with the monitor. The woman knew something was wrong. She told me she had not felt the baby move for a day. We tried to hold out hope to her while we listened for the heart, but I think she knew her baby had died.

I did a section on another woman, with Charlie, my chief for the day, assisting, and Carol in the room watching. She called later to tell me how great it had been to watch me working so competently. I knew what I was doing. I was in control. I could concentrate on the surgery and shut out the rest of the day.

In the afternoon I did a delivery with Tony Curry and he said he was amazed at the improvement in my skills. I did an episiotomy, as I was supposed to, and sewed it up.

Tomorrow evening I leave for Chapel Hill.

Tuesday   Day 65

I spoke in Chapel Hill and as usual, the speaking engagement was a chance for me to articulate my thoughts. It was wonderful and strengthening to feel connected with my former self: teacher, lecturer, home-birth attendant, women's-health activist. I spoke in the morning, and in the afternoon showed a videotape of a home birth I had done. I also met with the head of the family practice department in Chapel Hill who had just made a ruling that no physician in his department may attend a home birth. I certainly didn't change his mind, but I was at least able to discuss the issue with him.

The videotape was of a home birth in which I had spent much of the labor stretched out next to the woman, one hand resting on her abdomen, and doing the breathing with her. I haven't been that caring doctor here, the person who could be there with her patient so fully. It is as though that healing physician is still inside me, waiting to be retrieved again when I leave this training.

I arrived back in Everytown last night and called from the airport to say I'd be home soon. Heather said, "Mommy, Snuggles was hit by a car, but she's not hurt bad and they said you could pick her up from the hospital tomorrow." Snuggles had been hit a few minutes after I left Sunday afternoon and fortunately a neighbor took her to the vet. Sometimes I feel like a sieve trying to hold on to money.

Last Friday night I dreamed I was driving on a circular ramp with a metal railing. I remember bumping into it, but being bounced off the railing instead of going over. I was frightened but not terrified. I remember the relief of the railing catching the car and I remember thinking I had to slow down. This part of my life is all about climbing off elephants and about being caught and protected by metal railings.

Thursday   *Day 67*

I am trying to deal with the isolation of the hospital by bringing books to read and by trying to concentrate on learning as much as I can.

Fran returned from Los Angeles this week, and I kept pumping her for information about the American Public Health Association meeting, the National Women's Health Network Board meeting, and the panel where she replaced me as speaker on "Feminism and Childbirth." I miss that contact and most of the time I feel very isolated from the rest of the world.

Today I watched a delivery of Dr. MacDougal's. The woman hadn't had a baby in fifteen years and was overtly unhappy about this pregnancy. She started to go to pieces during labor, but then pulled herself together for the delivery. She was given epidural anesthesia and was having trouble pushing, and Dr. MacDougal kept yelling at her, "Push, push harder! Can't you push?" It seemed to me she had the knack of pushing but something was missing. I was reminded of the other woman who lost her power to push as the epidural became more effective. They teach that the epidural anesthesia doesn't affect pushing or the urge to push, but that's not what I am seeing. The woman kept trying but her power seemed drained out of her.

Friday   Day 68

I went to a school meeting Wednesday night and talked with Celeste, the medical student whose child is in Heather's class. She told me that the teacher is known for pushing children. She said, "Your child will never be pushed again as she is this year." Heather seems to be happy with school, but she is doing badly in her work. She should not be in first grade.

Yesterday I took Heather to buy fabric for a Halloween costume. She wanted to be a furry rabbit, but then she saw some soft white material and we picked out a pattern for a fairy-godmother costume. Heather has a passion for soft material. When she was two she always wanted to sleep in flimsy, smooth nightgowns. I'm looking forward to sewing the costume for her this weekend.

I've received a letter from a literary agent asking if I am interested in consulting on a book about women's health care. She said it would be a book, "not as radical as *Our Bodies, Ourselves.*" I think I am becoming even more radical than that book.

Sunday   Day 70

Yesterday was restorative. I went with Laurie and Fran to the Midwest Feminist Health Center's meeting. I am always torn between wanting a quiet day at home and my need to be with people with whom I can speak. Heather came along and found other children to play with. It was a quiet day and I mostly sat and sewed Heather's costume while members of the health centers discussed organizational and political issues. It is good to be reminded that so many people understand the care of women as I do.

My sense of peace ended this morning when I realized that Arlene did not come back at all last night. Last weekend she also didn't show up by Sunday morning. It is clear that this is not going to work out. I guess the question is whether I fire her now or wait until it happens again. I'll have to talk with Gail, since it will put a burden on her to see Heather off in the morning until I find someone else. Gail, a quiet, reserved woman in her forties, has been incredibly easy to have in the house.

Monday   Day 71

Arlene will be leaving. She is angry and sullen, and says she won't work weekends at all. I'm sorry, but she has been so distant lately there doesn't seem to be a way to negotiate. She will stay through this week, and I will advertise again.

Tonight I have to help Heather with her pumpkin for Halloween and I have to arrange for her to get a birthday present for a party she is going to tomorrow. In distancing herself from Heather and the house, Arlene has stopped all but the most essential tasks.

Karen Dole, the new part-time resident, will be starting tomorrow. Carol brought her to the floor today to meet everybody. Seemingly strong and certain of her opinions, she looks like someone who can take care of herself. Karen's arrival gives me more flexibility in my schedule: I will be able to leave at noon on the two days Heather gets out of school at one.

Wednesday   Day 73

I stayed and took care of patients on L&D instead of going to Grand Rounds this morning. While I was there alone, a woman came in with a baby who I thought was breech with a foot down. The woman had a section but I wasn't allowed to scrub on the case because this was another attending who is very old and is unofficially not allowed to operate without a chief scrubbed with him. I joked with him about Richard's having "stolen" the case from me because I didn't want him to realize why I had been taken out at the last minute. I don't think he knows that he isn't being allowed to operate alone.

Thursday   *Day 74*

Arlene left last night saying she would like to call Heather sometime. Another person is coming for an interview this afternoon, an ad will run in the paper this weekend, and I am posting a notice at the women's center. In the meantime, Gail will be getting Heather off to school in the morning. I will be home Tuesdays and Thursdays in time for Heather, and a teen-ager will be there the other afternoons.

Karen's arrival has in some ways increased my difficulties at work. Although I think we will be friends, still she is one more person like them and not like me. Richard told me, "Karen just knows how to be a resident better than you do. She knows the routines and procedures." Which means, she doesn't question them.

Sometimes I think, "If only Richard were gone, I'd be okay," but I know if it weren't Richard, there would be someone else like him. This system is designed for people like Richard to be successful.

I've convinced Larry Morris to take us on teaching rounds in the morning. He is a good teacher and I learn a lot from him. Going on his rounds, though, means that we have to be even faster on our own morning work rounds. I hate what I've become when I see myself make rounds in the morning and pass through efficiently, giving miserable care. I hate what I've become when I am anxious for Karen to hurry up and when I feel I have to tell her she can't be so careful and take so much time with each patient. It's a wicked program that destroys so much of what we are.

The support of my friends outside the program keeps me going. There's going to be a supper for the local NOW Health

Task Force at my house next month. I talked last night to the woman who is organizing it. I'm thinking of inviting Jackie and Carol but I feel there's still a gap between us because they are chiefs. It is painful that a separation exists between me and the other women, especially since I really like them.

Chapter Seven

The woman who was to come for an interview yesterday did not show up.

I arrived at the hospital this morning at six as usual, to see my twenty-two patients before eight, when I have to report to L&D. This morning I spent a few extra minutes with Maria, a sixteen-year-old who had a Caesarean section four days ago and was to be discharged today. Over the past three days I have enjoyed our brief morning encounters. I enjoyed the tenderness and delicacy with which she treated her baby. Teen-agers can be wonderful and loving mothers. It is the poverty and lack of support that create the problems, not lack of affection.

Maria loved to show me her little girl, to ask questions about baby care, but more than that, to look for my appreciation of her baby and the way she took care of her. Today she wanted to know if I thought her daughter knew her yet. Did I think the baby looked like her? This morning she had out the pink outfit the baby would wear for discharge. Each baby leaves the hospital that way, dressed up in pink or blue or yellow or white, packaged from the hospital with all the dreams of its mother's life, even the life of a teen-ager.

Maria had been standing over the bassinet when I came in, and now she slowly moved back to her bed, half bent, holding her abdomen with the palms of her hands, as though to keep her insides from falling out through her incision as she moved. This is a common position among women after a Caesarean and I wonder if they all worry their insides will fall out.

She had many questions for me, which I answered as I examined her and changed the dressing on her incision. Enders, her attending, had told me to remove the metal clips that held together the edges of her incision two days ago. I had unsuccessfully protested that it was too early and he had told me, "Remove them now. I want her out of here on Friday."

I gave Maria instructions on bathing, sexual intercourse, lifting, etc. I told her to make an appointment with the clinic in six weeks for both herself and her baby. Nervous about time and the difficulty I would have finishing rounds by eight, I said goodbye and wished her luck.

I checked in at L&D at eight to relieve Barbara and Beth, who were going off duty. Richard assigned me to follow a service patient, which meant he would be supervising me. I went to meet the woman, Angie Loren, thirty-two years old, mother of four, with some mild hypertension that had developed later in her pregnancy. She had been brought in at four this morning by her husband, who had gone home to take care of the others, and then would go on to work. Angie Loren was a quiet woman who seemed passive and accepting. She didn't demand much from me, and in a situation in which demands were often more than I felt I could carry, that was a relief.

Angie's blood-pressure increase posed a risk both to her and to her baby, so she was to be monitored closely. I examined her vaginally around nine o'clock and found her cervix about five centimeters dilated. She was becoming very uncomfortable and wanted anesthesia. I said we could put in the epidural catheter and wait until she was further along to give her the actual dose. I explained to her that if we gave her the medication now, we might slow or even stop her labor, but that later on, there was less risk of this happening. I went to the desk and called Anesthesia to come and see her.

The unit secretary called to me that I was wanted back on 3W, that someone was bleeding. I went downstairs to find that the edges of Maria's incision had separated and she had begun oozing blood through the opening of the wound. I called Enders and he said, "Marcelle, put on some steristrips and send her home anyway."

"But she's bleeding" was my futile protest. "She needs a packing."

I went back to Maria, who seemed remarkably calm, and I applied the small strips of adhesive tape to hold the edges together. I relayed the message that Enders said she was to go to the clinic in one week instead of six. I said goodbye to her again.

I returned to L&D to find that Angie was gone from her room. Sally, an experienced OB nurse who is going on to midwifery school, reported to me with a skeptical expression, "Richard came in and checked her and said she was only four centimeters instead of five, and therefore had made no progress."

"That's crazy," I said. "We both checked her and she was five."

"He said she needed x-ray pelvimetry so we could see if there was room for the baby to get through her pelvis."

I went out to find Richard.

"How come you sent her for x-rays?"

"She had an arrest of labor. Your exam was wrong, therefore her labor curve is off the norm. The protocol calls for x-ray pelvimetry, to see if she has CPD (cephalo-pelvic-disproportion) —when the pelvis is presumed to be too small for the baby."

"But her labor was just picking up."

Richard shrugged his shoulders and busied himself looking at a chart. I was angry. Angie hadn't been arrested to begin with. I knew I wasn't wrong in my exam, and neither was Sally. I was even more annoyed that I hadn't been part of the decision on a patient I was to be following.

Florence, another nurse with many years of OB experience, came out of the OCT room to ask for my assistance. "I've just tried and failed twice on an IV for a patient in the room, and there's another one in there with poor veins. Could you try?"

I didn't really have a choice, since I was the only junior resident around then. John was still in the back with a section. I agreed. It's not that I'm any better than she is, I'm just the next one to try. I have more authority and sometimes that helps. Maybe the veins listen to the person highest in authority.

The woman on the first stretcher had come in for the test as an outpatient. Her baby was overdue and the test was being done to determine whether to induce her labor or to go on waiting. Carolyn was friendly, and even apologetic about the nurse's difficulty in getting the needle into the vein. "I'm sorry you had to be called," she told me, "but my veins have never been good."

"Veins have a life all their own," I told her, only half in jest. "Sometimes they seem to be right there, and then you put the needle in and they seem to disappear. They're not very obedient."

I put the tourniquet around her arm, saw what looked like a small vein, and missed it. Apologetically I told her, "Sorry I'm not doing any better today. Let me try the other arm." This time I tried at the wrist. "This one looks good. Now all I have to do is to put the needle in the vein and keep it there." Carolyn seemed comfortable with this banter.

I looked at the vein and squinted my eyes as I felt it with my fingers and tried to "see" it with both my fingers and my eyes. I held it in place lightly with two fingers of my left hand while I slid the tiny needle under her skin and into the vein. Dark-red blood ran into the needle and up into the thin plastic tubing attached to it. "Don't move. It's in."

Florence took the tubing and attached it to the IV bottle, and taped the needle to the back of Carolyn's hand.

Mildred had been watching us intently from the other stretcher, and as I walked over to her she said, "I hope you do a better job with me than you did with her. I sure don't want you messing with my arm like you did hers."

I heard about Mildred when she was admitted two weeks ago. She has had medical complications requiring her to be on bed rest and on a special diet. She was hospitalized because she was unable to manage either diet or rest with five children at home. She was now being tested every three days with an OCT to see how the baby's heartbeat responded when her uterus was stimulated to contract with pitocin.

I had been aware of Mildred's watching me as I worked on Carolyn."I'll try to do better," I said. "Veins can be funny, though."

"You better not mess up, or I'll walk out of here. I'm so sick of people poking me and making mistakes on me."

"I'll try, that's the best I can do."

"You better do better than that."

I wanted to be able to stop the way this was going. She was getting me upset. I had put the tourniquet around her arm as we were talking, and now I saw that no veins popped up that I could see easily. I told her to squeeze her hand, and still none showed up.

"I'll try the other arm," I told her, feeling tension mounting and my own calm disappearing. As I squinted my eyes and felt her arm with the tips of my fingers, I questioned myself: Is that a vein or a tendon I'm feeling? My eyes see nothing, what of my fingers? Am I tricking myself? Why is this so hard sometimes and so easy at other times? I need to relax to do this well.

"Why are you taking so long?" Her question interrupted my thoughts. I understood her frustration, but I didn't want to be her target. I needed to finish in here and get out to see what had become of Angie Loren. I didn't want to be in this room.

I tried to get my balance, to remember who I was, why I was here, and why she was there. "I am not responsible for your being here," I told her.

She looked at me and in a flash I knew how she had heard my words. With horror I remembered all the doctors I had heard shouting at laboring women, "You didn't scream that way when it went in!" or "You should have thought of that nine months ago." The doctor examining a woman, trying to push his fingers into her vagina, yelling at her, "You had no trouble separating your legs nine months ago, did you?" The woman in labor screaming with pain, being told, "Why didn't you say no?"

I flashed on all the times women had been told that this pain and this abuse were their punishment for the crime of their pregnancy.

I had been thinking of this woman's medical condition and her domestic difficulties, not her pregnancy. I was trying to tell her and myself that I was not there to torture her, to inflict pain on her. I was trying to tell her that she was there because of her disorders, that they were the cause of her pain, not I. What she heard instead was the abuse that, for centuries, has been heaped upon women crying out in pain and vulnerability. I was now a part of that abuse.

The room was quiet. Then Mildred snapped, "You had no right to say that to me. I'm sick. I'm the patient. I can't help how I am."

"I didn't mean what you think. I wasn't even talking about your pregnancy. I meant I wasn't the reason you were here or needed an IV started." I was angry with myself, but the harm was done.

She was crying now. "I don't want you to touch me," she said angrily between sobs. "Let Florence try."

There was nothing left for me to do. I left her with Florence, a kind woman who would comfort her and soothe her.

I went back to the labor room to look for Angie, who should have been back from x-ray by now. Richard was there, hooking up the pitocin drip, which would stimulate her labor.

"She didn't have any CPD. There's plenty of room in there. I've decided to start her on pit."

He had read the x-rays while I was in the OCT room and had determined there was plenty of room for the baby to pass through Angie's pelvis. There never was any evidence that her labor had arrested. Within a half-hour her cervix was seven centimeters dilated.

I had to leave her room again to check a new patient who had come to the floor. When I returned, Richard was standing over Angie's bed with a partially opened fetal-scalp sampling kit. He said the monitor had shown questionable variations and he wanted to get a fetal blood sample from the baby's scalp to test in the pH machine. The pH of the blood is a measurement of the chemical balance of the body's metabolism. In obstetrics, the pH of fetal blood is sometimes measured during labor if the monitor strip shows patterns indicative of fetal distress. The blood sample is acquired by using a lance, similar to a finger lance, but on a long rod, to pierce the scalp of the baby in utero. The blood is then collected in long glass capillary tubes and is quickly run through the pH analyzer, a sophisticated, sensitive and sometimes erratic machine.

I told Richard I had watched the procedure several times now, and asked that he instruct me through the procedure on Angie.

"I've changed my mind. I don't think she needs it" was his response.

Angie quickly began to want to push. Richard did a vaginal exam and announced that she was fully dilated and would be allowed to push. Angie began to push, and with each contraction there were patterns on the monitor indicative of distress and I worried about whether the baby was all right. Richard told me not to worry, and left Sally and me with orders to take her back to the delivery room when she was ready.

I watched Angie and the monitor. When it was time to go to the delivery room, I decided to take the monitor back with us, since the pattern was still abnormal and she might not deliver for a while. Sally and I began wheeling her back, and sent a message to Richard that we were going back. Once there, I reattached the monitor and found that the heart rate was down to 60/min., less than half the normal rate. Richard came in and said to scrub.

We were out at the sinks scrubbing, looking through the window to the delivery room, when he said, "I want you to go back in there and turn off the monitor."

"But the rate was down to sixty when I left."

"I want that machine turned off."

I went back into the room, unhooked the machine, and returned to the sinks. I was furious. I had come to this hospital to learn the technology. It was what Richard is best at, and yet in my presence he becomes so antagonistic and oppositional, he cannot even teach me what he knows so well.

"I want the machine out of the room."

I went back again.

I returned to the sinks, scrubbed and went into the delivery room. Angie was screaming as she pushed. The baby's head was crowning. Sally and Richard were telling her to push harder.

I took the scissor in my hand to do the episiotomy, but Richard grabbed it from me and told me to do the delivery without the episiotomy. Ironically, I argued that I wanted to do one because I wanted to get the baby out as soon as possible.

We did the delivery with Richard looking over my shoulder, supervising. The baby's head came out without a tear, but there was a small tear when the shoulders came out. Richard continued to harass me throughout the sewing of the tear. He would tell me not to sponge up the blood as I was working, and to use my fingers instead of instruments, but then he wouldn't sponge for me either, so I couldn't see what I was supposed to be sewing.

The baby was okay, except for a high-pitched cry which is sometimes indicative of distress, and it had some irregular breathing at ten minutes. There was a lot of meconium as it was coming out and I would have liked to have a suction trap on the table, but I didn't dare ask Richard for one. We sent the baby to the nursery for observation.

While we were in on that delivery, I told Richard what had happened with Mildred, the hypertense patient, since I knew he would learn of it, anyway, and he told me to go back and apologize to her. I said I would go back and I would tell her I was sorry she was upset, but that I wouldn't apologize for what I hadn't said.

By two o'clock the woman I had admitted earlier was ready to deliver. Her attending didn't get there in time, so I was alone for the delivery. When it was over, the woman asked me, "Are you a midwife?"

"No, I'm a doctor," I told her laughingly. Her question had implied, "But you're too nice to be a doctor."

"She's really a midwife at heart," the nurse added.

"I guess I really am a midwife. It depends on where I am."

The nurses continued to joke about that exchange for the rest of the day.

The steristrips I had put on Maria's incision had not stopped the bleeding, and at two o'clock I was called back to see her. I asked Richard to take a look at it with me this time. He recommended that she be taken back to the operating room, given general anesthesia and sewn up again. He called Larry Morris, since by this time Enders had left for the weekend, and Larry said to start an IV and order blood in case she needed to be transfused. None of this was necessary but it helped legitimize her stay in the hospital. Larry finally came in to see her later in the day. He agreed we should put in a packing, which is what I wanted to do this morning. We did and it stopped the bleeding. I think she will be fine.

I went back to Mildred, who was by now back in her room, a large, gloomy place with three beds and curtains between them. I pulled the curtains which enclosed her bed.

"I'm sorry I upset you earlier." I was sorry she was upset but I wasn't sure I could explain myself any better than I had already.

"You had no right to say what you did." She was quickly tearful and angry again.

"I didn't mean it the way you heard it."

"You shouldn't have said anything. You're a doctor."

"You got me rattled, and I'm sorry that happened, but it did."

"Doctors should be able to take anything. Patients are sick."

"Well, that may be true, but I'm just another human being, and sometimes I get rattled."

"You shouldn't be that way."

I told her again I was sorry I upset her, and that I didn't think she needed to take abuse and neither did I.

It was by then four o'clock and I called home. The teen-ager who was baby-sitting told me Heather was playing with a friend outside.

L&D was quiet by this time. I told the nurses where I would be and then went into the doctors' lounge, put on the headphones and listened to a tape I had just received from my friend Ann in California. It was wonderful to be sitting in that room listening to the voice of a friend. Intermittently I looked over material from a woman's group I'm helping to write about childbirth. That work makes me feel needed and as if I have something to contribute.

Sunday   Day 77

As I drive in to work, Heather is home with my parents, who will take her to the zoo this morning. I woke at six, realizing I was late, but I was out of the house and in the hospital by six-twenty, and not missed.

This morning Dr. MacDougal let me do most of a postpartum tubal ligation. I hadn't been in surgery with him since my third week here, but was able to demonstrate my competence today. When he started to do something I knew how to do, I would tell him. He scrubbed out at the end, leaving me to finish alone.

I talked with him about Mildred, who is his patient. Richard had called Dr. MacDougal on Friday to tell him what had happened, but MacDougal's response this morning was that too much had been made of it all, that Mildred was a very difficult patient and that I shouldn't be worrying about it.

Yesterday I spent the entire day working on the health resource guides, which is work that feels as important a part of my move to Everytown as what I do at the hospital. My sense of purpose was reaffirmed as I was able to put my knowledge into words that would be read by many women. So often my being a doctor has made my thoughts suspect in the lay community, so it was exciting to find Fran and Laurie so receptive both to my opinions and my technical information.

Beautiful pink light is coming across the sky as dawn approaches. I won't see the sun come up because I'll already be at work, but it looks like the day will be beautiful outside.

I spent last evening interviewing women for the job of baby-sitter. Louise, a friendly young woman from Guadeloupe, impressed me most. I called a reference in New York and was told the children there still ask for Louise and wish she'd come back. She left there to be closer to an aunt here in Everytown. I've spoken with her aunt and her aunt's employer, who told me how responsible Louise is. I am reassured by her connection with this community. It is scary to take strangers into my house and have them be alone with Heather so much. The ordeal of interviewing again has involved meeting a number of restless women who are transient and have no roots. It's a strange life that causes them to go and live in other people's homes.

Heather is convinced that baby-sitters are hard to find because, as she puts it, "I think I'm a hard kid to baby-sit for."

"No, Heather, that's not true at all." I protested, suddenly surprised by her statement.

"Well," she said, crossing her arms over her chest and looking as if she had an important answer for me. "Arlene left because I was hard to baby-sit for."

"Arlene left because she didn't want to work that many hours. It had nothing to do with you."

I knew from her expression that she was not convinced. She felt responsible.

This afternoon, I met the infection control person for the hospital, and talked with her about the infection rate following Caesarians. She said our rate was about 30 percent, and that nationally it ran between 30 percent and 50 percent. The major cause seems to be the frequent vaginal exams and prolonged ruptured membranes. She added that the internal monitor may be a contributing cause.

The insulation man came to the house today to do the attic.

He apparently started to fall through and put a big hole in the ceiling of Heather's room. I've had arguments with him over the phone this afternoon, because I'm insisting that the ceiling be fixed.

I feel overwhelmed by the problem of looking for a housekeeper/baby-sitter, dealing with ceilings falling in, and exhaustion from my job. Today I dozed off for about half an hour while sitting straight up in a chair.

Wednesday, on the way home *Day 80*

I've requested a meeting with Dr. Pierce about a woman whose baby died in utero sometime last night. I admitted her yesterday with pre-eclampsia, an increase in blood pressure which is dangerous to both mother and baby. Because we were overcrowded on the floor and short of monitors, the nurse wanted to unhook this woman from the monitor. I refused to take her off the monitor, insisting that the baby was at great risk and we needed to find out what its condition was.

I had to leave the labor floor for a delivery, but when I returned, the pre-eclamptic patient had been moved off the floor. I felt there was nothing I could do because she had been moved to John's floor after both Richard and the attending had written orders on the chart to transfer her. After the baby died in utero, they looked at the monitor strip and discovered that it was evident yesterday that the baby was in distress. Richard has now complained to Dr. Pierce that I didn't follow the chain of command because I transferred her. I wish I hadn't adhered to the proper chain of command and that I had gone to check up on her. I hadn't liked the little bit of monitor strip I'd seen before I had to leave.

Last summer when I first met with Pierce, I had told him I could take orders. While I resent Richard's accusation and I need to clarify the truth with Pierce, I also wish I hadn't taken anyone's word that this woman was all right. In this scheme of things, though, human life is secondary to maintaining the system. My own ability to function here frightens me.

I've stopped to pick up groceries and guinea-pig food and litter. I'm almost home now.

Thursday   Day 81

"Michelle, I want to talk with you for a minute."

It was seven o'clock and I was in the middle of making rounds. I knew that Jackie, who was now the chief resident, wanted to talk with me about my meeting with Dr. Pierce. We went to a stairwell for privacy and sat on the top of the landing. Jackie's tension was evident as she ran her fingers through her curly black hair.

"I know Richard is difficult to work with, in more ways than you know."

I didn't ask what she meant. "Yeah, he gives me a hard time."

"In some ways you and he are the worst possible combination to work together, but you can't complain about him to Pierce. Pierce has to back his chief." Jackie's voice was tight and almost shrill. Tired from a long night of work, having been told she had the responsibility for whatever any resident did, Jackie was obviously worried about my meeting with Pierce.

I knew Jackie didn't want me to go to Pierce. A junior person isn't supposed to do that.

"I'm not going to complain about Richard," I assured her. "I'm going to tell Pierce that I haven't broken my agreement with him about following lines of authority. That was Richard's complaint about me and I have to answer him."

"Jackie, there's only one time I disobeyed Richard. That was the night he told me to go to sleep and instead I ordered a hematocrit and then awakened him with the results. He took credit for the test, and both of you took credit for saving the patient's life by taking her to surgery. I've never said anything about it. I know the rules."

Jackie seemed relieved and I think surprised that I was so cooled off about the issue. I guess someone told her how angry I was yesterday.

At our meeting I told Dr. Pierce, "It's like going to war and knowing in advance what you're going to be going through, but then finding yourself on the front line and not wanting to be shot at."

He laughed and said he liked my analogy.

I don't think Pierce had taken Richard's complaint about me seriously, because when I told him I had not broken my agreement with him about following orders, he said he knew that. We talked in general about how I was doing. I said I was happy that I had come here and that I never doubted that decision, although sometimes it was difficult on a day-to-day basis.

Pierce gave me some feedback. He said all my positive qualities had come through but that he had initially been worried about my surgical skills. I told him of my recent good experience with MacDougal and Black. "When they hand me the scissors in the middle of cutting the uterus, then I know I've convinced them of my capability."

"Well, if the old diehards are letting you do surgery, then you must be doing okay," he said and laughed.

I mentioned to Pierce a letter I had received about funding for research on cervical caps, a strong interest of mine before coming to Everytown, and I asked if his department was interested. I had been importing caps and fitting them in New Jersey. He asked if I was interested in doing research at Doctors on cervical caps, but I said I didn't think I could get involved in anything else now. He suggested that I not bow out so easily and that I mention to Lois Scott, their birth-control director, that there is money available.

Later Richard wanted to know how my meeting had gone. I shrugged and said, "Okay."

Friday   Day 82

Yesterday afternoon Heather and I walked downtown, bought groceries and walked back. She is having a tough time keeping up with the other children in school. Yesterday she asked me, "How many years do you spend in first grade?"

"Usually it's one, but if you haven't been to kindergarten, then sometimes it's two years in first grade and one in each of the rest."

"Will I be in Mrs. Nickle's class next year if I'm still in first grade?"

"I don't know that yet." Her teacher and I had talked about her repeating first grade and being in a K-1 with Mrs. Nickle. This conversation with Heather is painful to me. The whole subject is painful to me. Heather should have been in kindergarten this year and not first grade. I feel as though Heather is paying a heavy price for this move.

The meeting with Pierce has left me feeling much better about the program. I am pleased that he has not been dissatisfied with my work. I feel burdened by wanting to prove that having a part-time resident is feasible in a program.

Last night I received a call from a doctor in Washington who is interested in cervical caps. He said I may be asked to moderate a meeting in Washington of people from HEW, the Population Council, and the Feminist Women's Health Centers on research on cervical caps.

The cervical cap is a birth-control device similar to the diaphragm which has recently been reintroduced as a method of woman-controlled birth control. After reading about cervical caps in Barbara Seaman's book *Women and the Crisis in Sex Hormones,* I had begun importing them from England and using them on women who wanted to try them. The precise usefulness and statistical efficacy are still unknown, but the cap has become a political issue. Several days before I left for Everytown I learned that my last order of caps had been confiscated by the Food and Drug Administration in Philadelphia and that it would take a great deal of legal help to get them.

When I protested to the FDA officer in Philadelphia that "I spoke with the person in charge of Devices at the FDA in Washington, and she said it was legal for me to use them," he said, 'Well, she may tell you it is legal to use them, but she can't give you permission to import them."

Reluctantly, I agreed to having the caps returned to the manufacturer in England.

Today I spent a lot of time with Roberta, a woman who is in her ninth month and has been having some bleeding. She is a friendly person in her mid-thirties, pregnant for the second time. I examined her, and although there was nothing obviously wrong except for a small amount of bleeding, I was worried about her. The two most usual causes of bleeding in the ninth month are a placenta overlying the cervix (placenta previa) or an abruptio placenta, in which the placenta prematurely separates from the wall of the uterus. Both of those are dangerous conditions for both the mother and baby. Dr. Catan, her attending, ordered an ultrasound examination, which would locate the placenta, and I went with Roberta to the lab to watch the pictures on the screen. The radiologist decided they were okay and could find no reason for the bleeding.

I wanted Roberta to be monitored for the day, but Richard said no. I called Dr. Catan and by suggestion got him to say he wanted her on the monitor. Then I went back to Richard and said, with a shrug, "There's nothing I can do. Catan ordered the monitor."

Sunday   *Day 84*

Hilda Cameron and I had a long talk about the baby who died in utero earlier this week. Hilda told me she had never seen the monitor strip when the woman was transferred off the floor. The patient had been wheeled past her in the hall and she had asked, "But what about the strip?"

"It's fine" was the nurse's reply, and Hilda assumed someone else had read the strip. Her note on the chart that the strip was fine and that the woman could be transferred reflected what she had been told, not what she had observed herself.

Last night I dreamed my mother and I were at the shopping center looking at Hush Puppies because I thought they would be more comfortable on my feet. The reality is that my feet are terribly sore from my having to stay on them hour after hour. I've been wearing my running shoes, but even they hurt. Tomorrow I'm planning to get some comfortable shoes, the shiny kind, because it will be easier to wash the blood off them.

Louise moved in yesterday, giving me hope that it will be easier at home. She is wonderful with Heather, outgoing, cheerful, offering to read to her, play with her. Heather has latched on to her and has taken on the job of showing her around, telling her about the house, me, the pets . . .

On the way home

Nurses have usually been my friends. Contrary to the general belief that women doctors can't get along with nurses, there is often a woman-to-woman bond that can result in an easy and close relationship. Nurses and I have usually been allies.

There is a tension between me and the nurses here that I have never experienced before, and I don't understand why. I think it is partly due to my low position in the power structure. Richard is the chief of OB, and the nurses defend him. He flirts with them, though behind their backs he talks about how he can't stand them.

Then, too, I think the nurses are put off by how different my ideas are. I think they feel unappreciated by me because they believe totally in the kind of obstetrics they are practicing. They believe this is one of the best places in the country in which to have a baby, and they don't understand why I question so much, why I don't act as though this hospital is the best place there is.

Today they got mad at me because I didn't call ahead about a patient I was rushing up from 3W and they took out their anger on the patient. I had ordered some medicine for her severe vomiting, but instead of getting the medicine, the nurse went to make some private calls. There were six nurses sitting out in the hall just talking, and one on the phone and no one would help the woman who was vomiting.

The worst part of the isolation is that I begin to think, Maybe they're right. Maybe I'm all wrong about childbirth. I begin to doubt myself and to think I'm simply someone who can't fit in anywhere.

Wednesday   *Day 87*

I've probably done as many sections as vaginal deliveries this month. I like sections because I enjoy being away from the floor for two or three hours. The demands on me become limited by my being in surgery, and I can't be called for three things at once. Because sections are done with attendings, and my relationship with them is better than with the residents, I am free of harassment for a while.

Today I scrubbed with Dr. Owen, with whom I haven't worked since my first week here. The surgery went well and I impressed him with my abilities. I delivered the head, sewed part of the uterus, cut and tied the tubes, and finished the skin closure. The woman had become pregnant with an IUD in place, and we found the IUD in the membranes that surrounded the baby. Dr. Owen felt her uterus was too thinned out for future pregnancies, so after the baby was out, he said, "Doreen, I really think you should have your tubes tied."

Doreen was lying on the table, paralyzed from the abdomen down. Her husband stood at her head, holding her hand. "Why do you say that? You know I was thinking about it but had decided not to."

"Your uterus is so thinned out that I would worry about a future pregnancy. I want to tie these tubes now."

"Okay, I guess that decides it."

Then, addressing the rest of us in the operating room, he said, "We have decided to tie her tubes. I want you all to be witness that the patient has consented." She had not signed a consent for tubal ligation and I asked myself whether what we were doing was legal.

I tied both tubes, and when we reached skin closure, Dr. Owen left me to finish.

Sunday   Day 91

The blue sky is beautiful today. The days have been warmer than usual for November, so I am enjoying this bit of Indian summer.

My friend Missy is visiting from New Jersey. Yesterday we went out to Lake Animal Farm and enjoyed the animals and just being out in the country. Heather found a long rope swing to play on, and we all sat out on a blanket and talked. Louise is off for the weekend and Missy is taking care of Heather while I work today. This afternoon we'll probably go downtown to wander around and have dinner.

I am finally getting the knack of what they are trying to teach me. Ian Dorsi taught me today to have the woman stop pushing, and once I had control of the head and chin, to deliver the head myself without the woman's assistance. While this speeds up the process it is almost as though the woman is not there.

When I was delivering babies at home and even when I was practicing in South Carolina, the mother was the one who had control over what was going on. I never sought to take control, but worked instead at coordinating my hands with what the woman was doing.

Monday   Day 92

"Missy! I just realized why that delivery bothered me so much."

I had come home to find Missy knitting in front of the fire while Heather played with a friend. I sat and talked with her for a while but was then overwhelmed by a need to sleep. Now, two hours later, I awoke with a start, having reached an understanding in my sleep.

"The delivery of the head by the obstetrician reminds me of

159

men who boast of being able to make a woman come on command."

Missy said, "They like to be in control. No one challenges that control."

Later

My first patient this morning was Elise, a woman who had delivered at home last night and then came in because she hemorrhaged. It is uncertain why she bled because there was such chaos here last night when she arrived. The attending who was covering was so angry she had delivered at home with a midwife that he refused to come in to see her. The resident who examined her was never sure why she was bleeding, but it stopped.

This morning at six I went in to meet Elise, who had her baby with her, since a baby born outside cannot be kept in the nursery. I told Elise I had done home births and she seemed relieved to find a sympathetic doctor. She made up a story about who had been with her in order to protect her midwife. She said, "Some friends happened to stop by and they started an IV." I didn't press her for the truth because she needed to protect them, since they are practicing illegally. I enjoyed knowing that they were there, that they had taken care of her properly, and even that she was protecting them.

I heard in the afternoon that Elise was planning to sign out "AMA"—against medical advice. She was still being transfused and I didn't think she should leave. I was too busy on L&D to leave the floor and go to 3W, but I had her call me on the phone. She wanted to leave because she has a two-year-old at home, whom she is still nursing. I arranged for the little girl to be able to come in, and she agreed to stay until tomorrow. When I stopped down to see her for two minutes on my way out, she was in tears, having just put down the phone.

"What's wrong?" I asked. "Is it your baby at home?"

She nodded and then said, sort of embarrassed, "I just talked to her and she is fine without me." She was laughing and crying at the same time. I understood the feeling.

Tuesday   Day 93

It's still dark out and snowing and quite beautiful. Louise is working out so well at the house. Last night I came home, relaxed while Louise gave Heather her bath and then fixed supper for Heather and me, since Louise was going out for dinner. Then we ate some of the leftover ice cream sundaes, which were cold all through and reminded me of the old Good Humor sundaes I used to eat as a kid in New York. By eight-thirty I was in bed and asleep.

I told Fran on the phone yesterday that I felt as though the truths were being revealed to me about obstetrics, and I shared with her my new insights. I realize I never knew any of this before because I never had any close obstetrical supervision. When I was a student at City Hospital, I was simply left in a room with women about to deliver and I learned how to get the babies out without tearing. I fear I will lose that skill I developed naturally as I realize that what I do is so different from standard practice. I've had lots of people with whom to consult, but until now, no one has ever put their hands on mine and supervised me in the moment-to-moment delivery of the infant.

Later

Yesterday Tony Curry said to me, "If you can get Elise, the home-birth patient, to stay this one night, that's all I want. Once she's had her transfusions, I don't care when she goes home."

I had persuaded Elise to stay that day. Then, this morning Tony went into her room and she asked him when she could go home. When he didn't answer her, she said, "Dr. Harrison said I could go home today."

He became enraged at what I had told her—despite his instructions to me. In front of one of the nurses and a midwife, he said, "You cannot tell people when they can go home. You can only say to them, 'Dr. Curry will tell you when you can go home.'"

I was suddenly angry myself. The members of his group practice seldom saw their patients—the residents did all the work. "Dr. Curry, I've been told to treat your patients like service patients, and if that's not so, then you can see your own patients for postpartum care."

"Don't threaten me, Michelle."

"Well, I find it hard to get contradictory messages. If I'm doing all their care and you never see them, then I need to be able to tell them when they can go home."

"Well, just don't threaten me. You know we can do all our own cases." That was always the threat. They could take away our surgery. My mind spun off the answers I would have liked to give him, like, "I don't care if you do all your own cases," or "You don't want to do all your own cases, anyway, since you're a lazy bunch of doctors." However, I said none of those things, only "Okay."

I was surprised later when he came to me and said it had all been a misunderstanding. The midwife who was there told me later that he had asked her, "I was right, wasn't I?," and she said, "No, Michelle was. If you aren't going to see your patients, she has to be able to take care of them." There are some patients from his group who come and leave and never see their doctors.

Today at four o'clock Jackie sat down with those of us on OB and worked out the Christmas schedule. I will be off for three days at Christmas. I would like to go somewhere with Heather.

Wednesday   *Day 94*

This morning it is still dark and there is a fine snow falling to the ground. It is so peaceful.

Tomorrow is Thanksgiving and I miss my family, I miss a *sense* of family. I don't want to go to New Jersey, and I really wouldn't want them here. I feel too drained to deal with intense or close relationships, and superficiality is hard to achieve with close family—but I miss them, anyway.

Starting in January, I will be back on GYN and working nights again. I shall miss this freedom in my time and miss being home every night. I am already anxious about that schedule.

Sometimes I feel like an anthropologist at Doctors Hospital, where I study this strange culture of doctors and patients. Each morning I drive off to my field site, spend the time with the people there, and then dictate my notes of what I have observed as I drive home at night.

The great benefit of doing this training in Everytown is that I am not alone with the hospital culture, but rather that I am constantly provided with support and affirmation of who I am, by the community of friends I have here. Fran and Laurie, so often there for me themselves, have eagerly introduced me to their friends.

Later

Roberta, the woman who was bleeding last week, has lost her baby. Yesterday she had an ultrasound scan, which showed that the baby was dead. Today, in tears, she came into the hospital to deliver. We used prostaglandin suppositories to stimulate her labor, and then high doses of Valium and an epidural so she wouldn't feel anything. Extra Valium was used at the moment of delivery to put her to sleep so she wouldn't see the baby. I felt close to Roberta and wanted to be there for the delivery. I watched the dead baby, a little girl, come out.

Carol's patient Annette also delivered today. I had seen her once for prenatal care when Carol was sick, and she talked of wanting a homelike birth experience. I didn't tell her I had attended home births, but I was able to talk about her concerns. When I came in this morning Annette was in the Alternative Birth room, but her labor had stopped as soon as she was moved there.

Carol sent Annette for x-rays, which showed there was room for the baby to go through her pelvis. She then started her on pitocin to stimulate her labor. The use of the pitocin and the fact that the labor had stopped meant that Annette was no longer of low-risk category and she was moved back to a labor room instead of the Alternative Birth room. Annette's contractions picked up and she progressed slowly throughout the day. Carol asked me to stay with Annette while she made several trips to the OR for other patients. We kept hoping that Annette would deliver while Carol was with her, but then she had to leave for an hour to give a talk across the street. When she asked me to do the delivery, for then it would be as close to a home birth as possible, I felt caught in a dilemma because without Carol there I had no protection against Richard.

"Carol, I want you to know that leaving me here to do the delivery isn't a good idea. As you know, Richard and I don't do well together and I can't guarantee I'll be able to do it the way you want."

"Well, what am I supposed to do?" was her angry response to me as she left. I had thought that maybe she could get Jackie to cover the delivery, or someone else to give the talk. Later she came back and apologized for her outburst. She had wanted reassurance from me, which I couldn't give her because I had no control over the situation.

Annette's cervix dilated fully. The internal monitor would tell us if there was any sign of distress, so I felt we could take our time in getting the baby out and that Carol might even get back in time. The nurses kept urging Annette to push harder —they sometimes act as though a baby can't get out without the nurses' pushing. I said Annette could relax, push as she needed to. Her contraction would suddenly peak, and without any instruction she would pull up her legs and push as hard as she could. Then, for a while, Annette seemed uncoordinated and was having trouble pushing, and she said, "I'm not doing it right, I can feel that."

"Annette, I want you to try something," I told her.

The baby's head was now only about an inch inside her vaginal opening. I took Annette's hand and said, "Feel with me," as my hand guided her index finger to the top of her baby's head.

"That's your baby's head, right there and almost outside you."

I left her finger inside her vagina, touching the baby's hair, and went on, "Now, imagine a circle, a large circle. Flex your head, and your back, bring your bottom up, so your body is a semicircle, and now think about delivering the baby up and onto your chest." I demonstrated the circle formed by her curved neck, back and buttocks, and the path the baby would go to complete that circle and be on Annette's chest, in her arms.

Annette flexed her body, and on the next contraction the baby's head moved into sight. Annette pushed and then suddenly stopped and looked at me with terror.

"What's wrong?"

"I'm afraid the baby will tear out my insides."

After that, my main job was to tell her gently, "Don't be afraid, let your baby out."

By the time Carol was due back, that baby's head was visible even between contractions, I was doing perineal massage, and Annette was pushing well on the contractions. Carol walked in, came over to the bed, and on the next contraction Annette pushed the baby into Carol's hands. Her baby daughter gave a lusty cry and Carol placed her in Annette's arms. I think sometimes babies and mothers pick the moment for birth.

Friday   Day 96

Louise didn't come back from Thanksgiving at her aunt's house last night and this morning I feel like chucking the whole thing. Sometimes I think it isn't possible to do what I'm trying to do. Over the holiday Heather was weeping for the people she missed in New Jersey, and she was very upset and clinging to Louise when she left Wednesday night, crying, "You're not coming back, I know you aren't." I, too, have been missing New Jersey and the house and my friends there and feeling what Fran describes as the violence of this move. I feel strangely displaced, especially at holiday time, because my friends here are new and I miss those with whom I share a past.

Later

Louise called this morning to apologize for being late and for not calling. I am worn down by the strain of worrying.

A woman came into the hospital in very early labor and over the course of twelve hours she did not go into good labor. She was given a drug to help her sleep with the intention of stimulating her labor when she woke up. However, she was five centimeters dilated when she awoke and was quickly fully dilated. As soon as she began to push, the baby's heart rate slowed precipitously and stayed dangerously low while we prepared the woman for an emergency section. We also did a fetal scalp sample, showing a pH of 7.11, which usually means that the baby is in severe distress. Before we could do the section, though, the woman delivered vaginally and the baby seemed to be in perfect condition, breathing, crying and with excellent color. I don't understand the low heart rate or the low pH. I wonder if we know what we are doing.

Andy, my obstetrician and colleague in South Carolina,used to say, "Whenever I'm with a woman in labor and I feel like doing something, I go out in the hall and have a cigar."

Chapter Eight

Sunday, on the way home   *Day 98*

I was in the middle of a section today and suddenly I just wanted to be back in New Jersey. I wondered why I was here macerating women's uteri and how I could go on with this and why I had ever decided to do this to begin with. It was hard to stay in surgery in the midst of that flood of thoughts.

The woman today had a fine uterus, but we have rules that say she can only give birth in a certain way and she did not follow our rules, so we cut open her belly. But we cut in the wrong place and now she will probably never have kids again. Now she will probably have problems with intercourse. We have really ripped apart her insides and sewn them back together again, but they are not the way they were. The woman was so close to delivering and the baby's head was so far down that we had to have someone go under the drapes to push the baby's head back up into her uterus. When the lips came up I knew that at least the baby would be able to breathe until we got it out.

I was passively watching because this surgeon was doing almost all of the operation himself. And then while he was fishing around trying to put together the parts of the uterus, he said, "Something is wrong. You must have torn apart the inside lining of her uterus when you took out the placenta." That is when I freaked out because I thought I had been very gentle when

I removed the placenta. And that is when I realized I am putting my fingers in other people's bodies, and even when I am trying to be gentle I can do grave damage. I knew that something was terribly wrong because it didn't look like the inside of her uterus we were working on, but rather we seemed to be seeing the whole uterus, in one piece. The woman was awake and her husband was in the room, so it was impossible to talk freely about what we saw.

In the course of the next half-hour the surgeon discovered it was not that I had destroyed that portion of the woman's uterus, but that he had cut down in the wrong place and had separated the cervix from the body of the uterus. He muttered an apology for having blamed me, but that was of no help to this woman. Richard came in and tried to get the surgeon to get more help from Dr. Pierce, but the surgeon didn't want any help and in the end he probably repaired the damage as well as it could be done.

The woman had wanted to have natural childbirth. When it was evident she would be having a section her husband asked me, "Does this mean she'll have to have a section in the future?" Now this woman has been so badly torn apart she is probably not safe with any pregnancy, assuming she can even conceive. Then after surgery we all got together because the couple had brought champagne, and I had a sip of champagne with them and felt torn apart.

I hate this field. I hate these people. I hate all these babies coming out through holes in the belly instead of through the vagina. I hate it because this particular baby was in no distress, but the mother was tired from laboring and we told her there was an easy way out. The easy way out is that she may not be able to have more children.

We are doing something terribly wrong. I begin to think that the full dilation of the cervix is meaningless, that we may be telling women to push long before they should and thus wearing them out. It is true that the cervix dilates and then the baby comes out, but maybe it's not the cervix that has been slowing down the process. Maybe it's an entire process about which we still know little. We study how it happens and then we try to make it happen that way, but the whole framework may be wrong. Maybe even after some people dilate, there are still hours to go before the delivery. We set a limit of one or two hours of full cervical dilation and we say she must deliver within that time we have established after the cervix is dilated. We make women push all that time, even when their bodies do not tell them to push. We make them push until they are exhausted and then we tell them we have to take over because they are not strong enough to push out their babies. The second stage of labor is that time after the full dilation of the cervix and until delivery of the baby. It is an arbitrary distinction created by men. It is a construct. It may not mean that a woman can now push out her baby. Maybe pushing is all wrong.

Monday (my birthday)   *Day 99*

I am continually haunted by yesterday's surgery. Knowing the surgery wasn't necessary, I had such a sense of foreboding when we went in. We determine when the time has come. We respond to "maternal exhaustion" when we can't take it anymore. I'm not cruel; it's not that I want to see women suffer, but I don't know of a way to relieve maternal exhaustion without the possible loss of a woman's life, a woman's reproductive capability, a baby. We have not "cured" childbirth, nor are we on the verge, and yet for those of us who watch a laboring woman, it is a long and exhausting time and we feel called upon to offer help.

We were supposed to put this woman on an antibiotic study being conducted at this and several other hospitals, but with the help of the anesthesiologist we talked the woman out of being on the study. Even before the problems of the surgery she was a candidate for infection because of her long labor, the ruptured membranes and the many vaginal exams, all of which increase risk. If we had put her on the study, she'd have only a fifty-fifty chance of being given antibiotics, since she might get the placebo instead. Without the study, we knew her doctor would give her antibiotics, and with the subsequent difficulties in surgery, she will get large doses of antibiotics.

Several days ago I warned a woman she would have to be strong enough to resist our need to relieve her discomfort. She, too, ended up with a section. Her labor slowed and then x-rays were taken which showed there was enough room. She was sectioned, anyway, on the assumption that the x-rays just didn't show the tightness.

It would be good and it would be easy if I could just accept what they say and learn their protocol and do what they tell me to do, but I can't.

On the way home

"Dr. Harrison wasn't as brusque today."

"She just isn't someone you would feel you could talk to," a second voice responded.

I was standing outside a room, about to move the chart rack on to the next room, when I heard myself being discussed. The words of those women were painful for me to hear although I knew they were true. I had just left that room and those two patients were two of twenty-five I had to see this morning. They both have good attendings, who will see them, so I do little for them.

It's as though my time represents a reservoir of 120 minutes which I ration to twenty-five women each morning between six and eight. After the clerical and scut work gets done, I have about three minutes left for each woman, but answering their questions takes time. "When will the stitches dissolve?" "Do you think I should have a nurse when I go home?" "Will the doctor be in today?" "What can I do about my breast soreness?" "What do you think about breast-feeding?" "Dr. Harrison, do you have children?"

The questions are important, and should be answered. It is painful not to be able to respond fully, but sometimes I guess it is easier to discourage the asking than to have to say, "I can't talk to you now. I have to go on."

I feel that what I do in the morning is so futile that I am ashamed of it, feel it is not important. I forget what it is like for these women to be waiting for the doctor to come.

Hospitals infantilize people both because of their enormous power over individuals, and because people feel very vulnerable when they are ill. Even healthy people, once admitted to the hospital and put into short white open-backed gowns, act as though they were ill. Patients, frightened by the unknown facts of their particular conditions and by their lack of expertise, become afraid to ask, "What is my temperature? What is my blood pressure?" Afraid to offend, lest their care be affected, they accept passivity and name it trust.

Most of the morning was spent doing a section and tubal ligation with Fred Brooke, who complimented me on how well I was doing. I feel so comfortable doing sections.

This afternoon I admitted a woman who was having her fourth baby. She was requesting a tubal ligation to be done right after the delivery—a common procedure—but she didn't want any anesthesia until after the delivery because she planned to have natural childbirth. Her attending and the anesthesiologist wanted to give her the epidural anesthesia for the delivery to save themselves the time that would be "wasted" between the two procedures. They said, "If we wait until after the delivery for the anesthesia, then it's considered an elective procedure and we won't do it now."

In the midst of the woman's cries of agony and insistence on natural childbirth, the nurses put her on her side and held her in place while the anesthesiologist tried to get the needle in place. When the resident failed at the epidural I had to leave the room. He had already failed on the section patient this morning.

The attending followed me, angry that I was not urging the woman to have the epidural.

"I'm not having anything to do with pushing someone to have surgery they aren't sure they want," I said, "especially a tubal ligation. She seems ambivalent about the whole thing."

"She's a patient in the Health Maintenance Program and we

can't afford the extra hospital days it would cost for her to have the surgery done later," he answered angrily.

The woman became fully dilated as we were talking. I ran back and delivered her on the stretcher before we could get her onto a delivery table. The baby had a lot of fluid in her throat which I suctioned out, and then I handed her over to the anesthesiologist, who by then had arrived. He put a laryngoscope into the baby's throat in order to show another resident how to look, and each time he did, the baby's breathing and heart rate slowed down considerably.

The nurse, who had been impatient with the woman's uncertainty about surgery, said angrily to me, "She's ambivalent, that's why she isn't cooperating."

"That's precisely why we shouldn't be pushing her," I agreed.

"I think she's confused and that's why she's willing to put it off."

"All the more reason we shouldn't be doing it now." Everyone was furious at this woman because of her uncertainty. In the end she said she would have it done some other time.

A Greek woman who needed postpartum instructions met with me and an interpreter for about a half-hour to talk about care of herself and her baby. The baby is jaundiced, so he will not be going home today and the woman will be allowed to stay too. I read once that jaundice comes in waves and we seem to be in one now, or else I'm much more aware of it now.

The nurse came in and told her how to take care of the baby's circumcised penis. She whispered to me that she describes it like Carvel ice cream in telling people how much vaseline to squirt on the end of the penis. The mother seemed upset about her baby. Later I was on 3W and saw the woman and her husband standing looking through the windows of the nursery at their baby now wrapped under the bili-lights, which are used to treat the jaundice. At three days of age the baby has had the tip of his penis cut off and will spend at least twenty-four hours under purple lights with blindfolds around his eyes.

Late in the afternoon I stood and looked out the window at the snow and thought about my birthday, and wrote some notes for some poetry. I thought about how much Heather wanted it to snow on her birthday. I called her at four just to say hello, but she wasn't home.

I thought about Saturday night when I was visited by Fran, Laurie and Serena, her mother, and Catherine, who all arrived for a surprise birthday party which Gail had worked hard to put together. My worlds are so separate from each other.

Wednesday   *Day 101*

Seven of the twenty-one postpartum patients on 3W have had sections. Several of them are infected. This morning I decided to miss teaching rounds and instead to spend time taking better care of these women, which meant missing part of Grand Rounds. I can joke or laugh about patients saying I'm too brusque, but it does bother me inside, and I guess it should.

Yesterday afternoon, however, Larry Morris took me aside and said,"You're doing very well here, but talking too much with patients is a problem you have." He was being friendly and supportive as he added,"I'm sure you'll learn to correct it!"

I went on to Grand Rounds, where the last speaker was from the School of Public Health. He spoke on nutrition in pregnancy and when we talked after the meeting, we realized we knew each other from a maternity-care conference in which we had both participated. His talk today was exciting, but was met with general hostility by the attendings, who tend to disregard any aspect of pregnancy except drugs and intervention. There is also a bias among doctors against those who do not practice clinical medicine, and especially those in public health. It is as though "real doctors" are the ones who do something with a patient. Especially among surgeons, everyone else is suspect.

I'm finding it difficult to have someone in the house whose job is to help us clean—without Heather then expecting to be waited on. Louise does much more for Heather than I want her to and I think it will take a lot of talking to get a better balance.

For all that, though, I'm worried that Louise may leave because I overheard her on the phone last night talking about what sounded like a strong pull to return to Guadaloupe.

Friday *Day 103*

There's a beautiful star in the east, not like any star I've seen before. It's morning, still dark, and I don't feel as if I've slept at all.

On the way home

I used forceps today. I was petrified as I put on the blades and pulled that baby out. The baby has a mark on its cheek, which I hope goes away. The advantage of attendings who don't care about their patients is that I get to learn more.

Yesterday on rounds I saw a baby with a cut on its face and the mother said, "My uterus was so thinned that when they cut into it for the section, the baby's face got cut." The patient is always blamed in medicine. The doctors don't make mistakes. "Your uterus is too thin," not "We cut too deeply." "We had to take the baby" (meaning forceps or Caesarean), instead of "The medicine we gave you interfered with your ability to give birth."

Sunday *Day 105*

My mother and sister are back at the house helping get ready for Heather's birthday party this afternoon. I'm hoping to get out a little early today if it isn't very busy.

Heather has been especially excited by the visit of my sister and my ten-month-old niece. Heather has always loved babies. She is gentle with them, as she is generally with everyone. Heather was very upset about leaving her cousin Abigail when we moved, and has now had a chance to spend hours with her, talking, making her laugh, showing her toys. Heather is even better than some adults in relating to babies as real people while also recognizing the limitations of their age.

On the way home

A woman came in today twenty-seven weeks pregnant, bleeding and in premature labor. This is her third pregnancy: her first was a section, her second a vaginal delivery. Both babies were premature and tiny. She has been told she has an incompetent cervix, one that opens too early and too easily, but which in her case cannot be repaired. She has been on bed rest the past couple of weeks because the sac with the baby has been bulging through her open cervix. When I admitted her I discovered that the baby was also breech, and its tiny feet were protruding through the membranes.

We hooked the woman up to the monitor, although no one was sure why, since we hadn't yet decided if we would do a section to deliver the baby. Charlie, the chief for the day, called in Richard, who called in Jackie, who called Larry. The woman's husband said, "We want everything done that doesn't jeopardize my wife." They had never been told that a section does jeopardize a woman. Even though he didn't understand the choices, the husband's statement became the deciding factor in delivering the baby by section. The tiny baby girl, a little over one pound, is not expected to live. As in any section done for fetal distress, "saving" this baby might have been at the expense of the mother.

I didn't get out early, but I'm heading home now to my family and Heather's birthday party. The transitions are difficult. Sometimes I wish I had more time to travel between work and home, time to let the day be absorbed, and to be alone with my thoughts.

Monday   Day 106

I made it through the beginning of school, through Halloween, through Thanksgiving, and now through Heather's birthday. This morning when I got to work I realized I had forgotten to bake cupcakes for Heather's class party today. I was in a panic until I remembered Louise. When I called her, she agreed to pick up cupcakes at the bakery and bring them to school for me. I called home this afternoon and found that it had all gone smoothly. I think there is a part of me that is so defensive about being a single parent and working mother that I drive myself to be sure my kid gets everything the others do.

This morning, arriving on L&D, I met Neil Anderson walking out of a labor room, his brow furrowed, and muttering, "I hate patients like that! I can't stand taking care of them!"

"What's up? Who is she?" I asked.

"It's one of those couples who obtained signed agreements in advance stating exactly what they want and don't want. Her husband is hovering over her and won't let me touch her."

"I'll be okay with them," I told him rather flatly, concealing my pleasure with such patients.

I walked into the room to see the woman laboring, her husband at her side, and another woman stroking her arms and coaching her. I introduced myself quietly and the coach said, "Yes, I've heard of you. You're from New Jersey, aren't you?" I recognized her instantly as someone with whom I felt a bond, someone who spoke a language of childbirth similar to mine. She told me her name, Nancy Carr, and said she worked as a private labor coach to women giving birth in the hospital. A warm and gentle person, she provided a support reminiscent of a home birth.

Neil came back and I was able to run some interference for the couple, especially in their not wanting an episiotomy.

Nancy and I kept telling Neil how well he was doing, so he was able to get through the delivery without doing an episiotomy and without getting too angry about the obvious pressure on him.

After the delivery Neil, in an inquiring way, said, "Michelle, why don't women like episiotomies?"

"Because it feels like a violation."

"That's ridiculous," said Rennie, another attending in the hall. "It's important to do them. Don't women understand they will stretch too much if they don't have one?"

I try to stay cool and detached for these questions, especially since I don't think my answers are heard. "Well, Neil, first of all, it has never been proven that they would stretch more. Second, it's painful after the delivery, and third, you asked why women don't like them and I'm saying that many women feel they're being mutilated without having any choice in the matter."

"But if you explain why it's necessary . . ." he protested. In medicine there is the belief that if a patient doesn't do what the doctor has suggested, then the doctor just hasn't explained the matter enough.

Feeling frustrated, I tried saying it a different way. "Look, I don't think it's something men can understand, even sensitive men. It's like you can't explain what pre-menstrual tension feels like, or childbirth—or even rape. It's something that is unique for a woman."

Neil was taken aback, and he protested angrily, "You know, my car was broken into recently and I had feelings that were like those of being raped, so I do understand the feelings of women who are raped."

I regretted having gotten into this discussion. "I don't want to argue with you. You asked me how women feel about episiotomies and I'm telling you."

We talked a bit more and they wanted to know about perineal massage, the method used by midwives to keep a woman from tearing during a delivery. "Tell me about it," Rennie said.

I'd been thinking a lot about what doctors do to women and

177

I responded, "I'm afraid to teach you guys how to do it. You'll come up with a perineal massage machine and women will be screaming while they get their vaginal openings ironed out with it."

They took my response as a joke. Rennie, intrigued by what I was saying, told me, "I have a cousin in New York who is a feminist."

I did two more deliveries with them and then a tubal ligation with Tony Curry, who let me do the case.

I stopped on the way home to look at TV sets, having decided finally to get one. I gave up television when Heather was a baby, but I agreed to get one as part of this move to Everytown, partly I think as a replacement for me. I'm caught now in a dilemma about what kind to get, whether to get black-and-white or color. Heather wants a color set because they're nicer to look at. I'm concerned about safety and radiation from color sets. I also worry about spending money to "buy" away guilt for not being home with her more. On the other hand, I don't want especially to deprive her, at least not for the sake of deprivation. I looked at several sets and I'll have to think about it more overnight.

With so difficult a year, I get upset with myself for getting embroiled in issues like which TV to get. I feel so drained from work, I seem to be missing some resources with which I usually make such decisions.

Tuesday   *Day 107*

There is a new paper out on the benefits of ambulation, or walking, during labor. I brought it to L&D and left it there for people to read, but then I realized that the problem is one of control, not method. I suddenly saw obstetricians deciding everyone should ambulate, and I saw women being forced to march up and down the halls while in labor, and doctors—men and women—standing there with whips ordering them to march on because "It's best for you." It's "them" deciding how "we" are to labor. We are left to argue with one another about how we should be forced to labor, to give birth, to raise our children.

Last night at dinner, Heather and I were joking with Louise about what a wonderful person she was to have in our lives. I told her I'd never in my life been so well taken care of, and then told Heather that Louise was my baby-sitter too. Louise laughed and said she was very happy here.

Heather has been in a wonderful mood the last few days. She's eating well, likes celery, which last week she hated, and is generally easy to live with. She's also doing better in school, and is finally in a reading group.

I've decided on a color set. Heather says, "Big Bird has to be yellow, and Grover has to be green." Maybe this afternoon I'll have a chance to look up *Consumer Reports* and decide which kind to get.

This afternoon I have to get a new driver's license, since my New Jersey one has expired without my realizing it.

Yesterday I received a call from a doctor in California who was looking for curriculum material on women's health care. If she can get funding, she will invite me out there to do a workshop. She told me that the American College of Obstetrics and Gynecology requires only one year of OB for a family physician to have Caesarean-section privileges at a hospital. I must also do twenty-five sections during that time. Since I am in a part-time residency, I would need about a year and a half in a program. Still, that would allow me to do my own sections as part of an OB practice. I must remember to document the sections I do.

Nancy Carr, the labor attendant, was in with another patient, and supporting her through a difficult labor. Irv Warren, the attending, was also determined that the woman would get through without anesthesia because, being over thirty, she will have a "premium baby." Besides, she was infertile for some time, so he wasn't taking any chances.

With the help of a very supportive nurse today, I managed a delivery without an episiotomy, worried all the time that Richard or the attending would show up and be angry. I was actually going to do the episiotomy, but Vivien, the nurse, encouraged me not to. The baby was fine and he cried before his body was fully out. I put the baby right onto the mother's chest instead of clamping the cord first, which is how I always did it at home. The young black woman and her husband were thrilled with the delivery. I'm always excited when I can provide that kind of experience for black women, because they rarely get good treatment in the hospital. Even middle-class blacks are treated differently from white women.

After the delivery I thanked Vivien, the nurse, several times. She gave me a hug and said it was wonderful to have me here. I wouldn't have been able to do it today without her.

Friday   *Day 110*

Next Tuesday I'm going to a lecture and slide presentation on giraffes and their style of mothering. They apparently give birth in isolation, but when their young are about two weeks old, each mother finds other mother giraffes with babies and they team together and create giraffe kindergartens. The mothers take turns staying with the babies while others go off for food and water. If there is danger, the mother left behind takes all the young to safety or protects them all.

I'm looking forward both to the lecture and to the time I will have wandering by myself around the university. I miss contact with poetry and music. I keep saying I have to do more, but I don't know where that energy will come from, since it's hard after the hours of work and child care to provide anything for myself except sleep.

I've been thinking about the ACOG requirements for sections, and my need to document more. I realize I have to push for more sections and not give them away as I have done, often preferring to watch patients in labor. I have the feeling that at night the residents want more surgery and do sections under circumstances they would take the time during the day to observe longer before deciding on surgery. They often operate for arrest of descent of the baby, but one third of those arrests are the result of their own intervention, the epidural anesthesia. Often the attendings also prefer sections because they are over with sooner, and the doctors can go home to sleep or start the day.

Later

Enders mumbled throughout the section this morning and I kept saying, "Excuse me, sir, I can't hear what you are saying." He still got angry each time I couldn't do what he wanted because I couldn't hear him. He still calls me Marcelle, although by now I am sure he knows my name.

Jerry Lambert is a young attending who let me help him do a delivery this morning without an episiotomy. He even let me hold back his hand as he was trying to stretch the perineal tissue when I knew it should be supported instead. Late this afternoon we had a long talk, during which he commented that I seemed to be more interested in learning and in patients than I had been when I began the OB rotation. I knew at the time that Jerry and others thought I was uninterested when, in fact, the problem was Richard's refusal to teach. Jerry had been especially distressed last month about a patient on whom he wanted x-rays. That was the day I was unsuccessfully trying to get Richard to teach me how to read them. Jerry had interpreted my inability to read them as lack of interest. Later I was sorry I had spoken so openly with him, since I heard him repeating what I had said to Richard. I'm also sorry because talking with him stirred up my need to talk with people here.

Chapter Nine

I've put up a year-at-a-glance calendar on my bedroom wall and it makes the whole year seem shorter. Six months is only six months away, and is made up of little units, each of which I seem, in some way or other, able to survive.

I'm on my way to work in the deep snow, having dug out the car and scraped it, and congratulate myself on having snow tires. It doesn't seem like much, but it makes me feel on top of what I am doing.

Each time we have moved, Heather has missed the friends she left behind. She was only two and a half when we went from South Carolina to New Jersey, but for months she would wake up in the middle of the night crying for Harvey, a four-year-old friend. I would find her in her crib, shaking the rails, calling his name as if she could bring him back or make him appear as he must just have been in a dream. She spoke of wanting to go to South Carolina and, in fact, remembered everyone the following year when we visited.

Heather's closest friend in New Jersey was Andrea, a girl who lived across the street, but whose father lived in Everytown. Heather, who had initially "refused" to move from New Jersey because she didn't want to leave her friends, was thrilled this week when Andrea came to visit. She will be back here for Christmas, too, so the girls will be able to spend time together.

Heather has been happy coming home in the afternoon. She spends her time playing independently in the neighborhood and is pretty responsible about letting someone know where she is. Aside from bike riding, though, the girls here tend to sedentary play. I wish I could get Heather interested in some active sports. She once told her grandmother, "Girls don't run," and in a game with her grandfather she insisted that she play the nurse, he the doctor, explaining, "Boys are doctors."

On the way home

This morning I made rounds, scrubbed on a section, did a tubal ligation, and then fought with Jackie about the next GYN rotation, which starts in three weeks.

"Michelle, I'm not prepared to pick up the slack for your being part-time," she began.

"What are you talking about, Jackie?"

"I don't want to be in the position Richard is in of covering for you. He's had to take care of patients on 3E." Her beeper went off and she left before I could respond. No one had ever suggested that I take care of patients on 3E. I did some work on the floor, checked a patient, and by then Jackie had returned. She only reluctantly let me have the rest.

"Richard has been telling everyone that it is difficult to cover the service because of your being part-time and not being able to finish your work." I pointed out to her that in the past two months the bed capacity of 3W had increased by five more patients and that my being part-time had nothing to do with making rounds in the morning.

"Well," she went on, "I'm making the schedule for the next rotation when I'm going to be your chief. I don't want to resent you, Michelle, and the only way I can prevent that is if I don't have to carry any of the load."

My frustration and resignation were mounting. "Jackie, I frankly don't care if you resent me or not because there isn't any way I can do everything." I reminded her that she had two part-time people at two-thirds time instead of one person, so she had even more help than usual.

"I want to like you," she said in a both whining and pleading way, then added, "and I want you to like me."

Jackie mentioned again, as she had the first day I spoke with her, that her husband had known a part-time resident who hadn't done *her* share of work. Once again she told me she would choose to have an abortion rather than be a resident with a child. She went on to say there was a lot of resentment about my being part-time. They're all so overworked that it's natural for them to object to anyone working less than they are. I told her I understood but was prepared to live with that resentment, since my only other choice was to quit and I wasn't going to do that.

Part of Jackie's problem is that Barbara, who is assigned to the abortion service for the next three months, doesn't do abortions on principle, so the rest of us will have to cover for her. I suggested that Jackie should be angry with Barbara instead of with me.

Karen Dole called me at home late in the afternoon to say Jackie had just told her she'd had a terrible fight with me, but that something else had been on her mind unrelated to me. Karen and I talked a long time about the schedule and how we could best share the time. Heather fell asleep while I was talking with Karen and didn't wake up until evening when I was leaving for a party. She cried because I had promised I'd make popcorn with her. For the first time I explained to her that I'd had a bad day at work and that I'd been so upset that I found myself talking about it at home and that's why I'd been on the phone. I'm not sure if I should tell her, but it may give her some insight into the reasons why I'm sometimes distracted and far away.

Monday   *Day 113*

Last night's party was in celebration of the opening of the new women's health center here in town. It was wonderful, though, and I met people of whom I'd heard but never met. I met two women who are studying at the School of Public Health and wished I could join them for lectures sometime. I miss intellectual stimulation at work. There seems to be no one grappling with anything except the uterus and its contents. Just as important, when I'm with my friends I feel a warm response and validation that I only feel at work from the patients—almost never from my colleagues.

Later

Today, as I was sewing up a woman's episiotomy, I thought about how much more I know now than three months ago. I have to keep sight of how valuable this training has been.

I am more and more bothered, though, by the "pushing" we force on the laboring woman. Today I walked out of a room in which Alice, one of the nurses, was yelling and yelling at the woman to push harder. Alice welcomed me to the floor when I first arrived, but now I find her one of the hardest to take because of the force she applies to women. I find myself hanging back and underestimating the dilation of the cervix on her patients because I don't want that intensive pushing to start. She makes the birth a hysterical event, as though the baby wouldn't come out unless she yelled.

Tuesday   Day 114

I stopped on the way home last night and bought a small color TV, which was an instant success. I sat and watched with Heather for a little while.

Heather has been in a wonderful mood lately. Last evening as we watched TV I felt she was trying to be very "grown-up" and have an earnest conversation. She has "definitely" decided she will be a teacher when she grows up. She also wants to be a "candy striper," which she interprets as someone who gives out candy to sick people, and a vet because she loves animals. I think she'd make a good actress!

She and her friends have been covering themselves with Heather's birthday make-up. Arlene, the baby-sitter, was always heavily made up and Heather at six is trying to emulate her. Heather has always loved make-up, though—and dressing up—and playing with dolls with an intensity I never experienced. At two she was already dressing herself, insisting on choosing what to wear. It was strange to realize how different she and I were. She cannot pass a shoe store without picking out several pairs of shoes she "always wanted."

I bought her the make-up hoping she'll get it out of her system during her childhood. I also bought her some skin cream, which she is enjoying. Since she was a toddler, Heather could be trusted to leave anything alone, including cookies or candy—except skin cream. She had no self-control, and if she found any, she would cover her body with it. When I was angry, she would look at me apologetically because she really couldn't help herself.

After a quiet evening at home with Heather, I find myself thinking it would be a blessing to be kicked out of the program in July.

Wednesday   Day 115

Those who hold babies and bathe them and feed them in their first days should be loving people. I doubt that the question is asked of nurses who apply to work in nurseries, "Do you love babies?" Mostly it is a matter of finding people who "aren't bothered" by the crying of infants.

The woman who delivered last week with Nancy Carr's support has written a letter thanking me for being "sensitive and humanistic." She especially thanked me for the way I introduced myself to her. She had been in the midst of a contraction when I walked in, introduced myself and said, "You don't have to open your eyes. I just want you to know who I am." She then felt reassured and confident that I knew how she was feeling and that everything was going well. I remember that moment because I thought at the time that as the doctor in this setting, I'm supposed to have the patient acknowledge me, pay attention to me. Yet that attitude went against my grain. It was good to hear that I had done what I ought to.

I stopped in the nursery today to look at a baby who was being delivered just as I went home yesterday. He has huge swelling and paralysis of the face from the forceps. The doctor who delivered him went through a uterus last week and cut a baby, and in another section a baby ended up with a fractured arm that no one can understand.

Today I worked with Jackie and realized that she is being trained to see every patient as an OB-GYN history, that for her every female must represent an onset of menstruation, pregnancy or nonpregnancy, birth control or no birth control. I fear that is what I will have to do if I am to succeed in this field, but I like to look at the women first, and wonder about them. That seems more important than training yourself to see only their illnesses.

Thursday   Day 116

Louise said last night, "I'm going away Saturday, for Christmas."

I was surprised, since Christmas is still two weeks away. I immediately tried to figure out how much this was going to hurt. "When will you be back? I really need you here."

"I'm going to Guadeloupe for Christmas. Afterwards I'll return." She seemed uneasy. I had a feeling I wasn't hearing something, or understanding something.

"Louise, when are you sure you will be back?" She was quiet, looking away from me, and I asked, "Are you coming back?"

"No," she said in one soft word that suddenly brought dozens of thoughts flooding into my mind, like Why is she leaving? Can I persuade her not to? What will I do about Heather? Gail is away until mid-January and she is tired of doing child care. I can't ask her anymore.

I thought of my few hours alone at the university this week and knew that the first thing to go would be any time for myself. I had even thought of having Louise work part of the time when

I was home at Christmas, since it would be nice to have her taking care of Heather and her friends while I relaxed. Instead I will be worrying about dishes and laundry and garbage and keeping the house a little bit straightened up, and wishing I had a few minutes to read or answer some letters.

Louise and I talked more. Between my tears and rage, I learned the full story. She has an aunt in Guadeloupe who has power over her and has told her she must return. Louise cried because she said she wanted to stay but she is afraid of her aunt. She agreed to stay until a week from Saturday instead of leaving in three days.

In my tears, I was also furious with Jackie for treating me as though I were lazy and for not understanding the real energy that goes into keeping my home afloat. The problem is that no one respects my work as a mother. If I were doing important work for NASA, the others would still resent my being part-time, but they would understand and respect what I was doing.

Later

It was impossible to talk with Jackie without crying as I told her I was having trouble keeping everything together, that my baby-sitter was leaving, and that I couldn't work past five-thirty on my next rotation, since the teen-ager has to be home by six. So, I've now traded my few free afternoon hours for the half-hour or so between five-thirty and six. My day will be only eleven and a half hours instead of twelve or twelve and a half. I'll still be working every fifth night as part of the night-call schedule.

This evening I tried to take a nap but couldn't, because I lay in bed thinking about a woman who was almost sectioned today. Dr. Owen had told her she might need a section. Visibly upset, she replied, "No, I don't want one."

"I'm sorry, dear," he said, "but we might have to section you, anyway, if that seems the best thing to do." Later, after the delivery, her husband said to her, "If we had decided you needed one, it wouldn't have mattered if you said no."

My left foot won't stop shaking as I drive. Dr. Pierce wants to see me in his office, but I couldn't get off L&D to meet with him and now I'll have to wait until Monday. I have no idea what it is about, but I am more and more worried as I become aware of my differences with the methods of hospital childbirth.

Today another woman came in wanting natural childbirth, and then asking for pain relief and a sedative—which she was given. The anesthesiologist wanted to put in the epidural needle, but we hadn't yet gotten a monitor tracing on the baby because no machine was available. I objected to giving the medication before we have a tracing, since it gives a pattern similar to fetal distress.

"It's too early to place the epidural," I argued. I remembered Dr. Warren's patient with the "premium baby" and his refusal to give her anesthesia because he didn't want to do anything to jeopardize that baby.

Karly, the nurse, argued with me, "Well, does that mean you wouldn't ever give an epidural?"

"I'm not thrilled with them, because of the fetal distress I've seen, but I definitely wouldn't give them to a woman who's already had fetal distress."

"But we don't have a free external monitor, so we can't get a tracing unless you rupture her membranes and get an internal monitor tracing. That's what you should do." The nurses, who are used to residents coming through for a few months at a time, year after year, are also used to telling them how to take care of patients. Usually they are less direct, though.

"I don't want to rupture membranes," I explained, and at the same time clarified for myself. "Once we give her the epidural, there is a good chance we will end up with an arrest of labor of some sort, and then doing a section." I was finally getting to say out loud the sequence I often repeated to myself. "If I have to rupture membranes now, and put on the internal monitor, then by the time we do the section she will have a higher chance of infection because of her ruptured membranes."

The anesthesiologist was standing there impatiently, so I turned to him and said, "If you want to put in the catheter, you can call Richard and I'm sure he'll overrule me, and that's fine. I just can't do it to her." Then, turning to Karly, I said, "Maybe tomorrow I'll be able to write an order like that again, but I can't today."

Karly walked away angrily, obviously in disagreement with my position, but came back later in the day herself in tears, telling me, "I can't stand it! I can't stand it!" An attending had come by and ruptured the membranes of a woman in very early labor. Karly knew the woman should have been left alone. Sobbing, she told me, "I can't stand their always messing people up. Why can't they just be careful and leave women alone to labor as they should?"

Last week there was a woman who wanted an epidural. Once we told her that she couldn't have one because we thought her baby was in danger, she coped beautifully with the pain. It's when you know there is no relief that coping becomes possible. Maybe that's the secret of how I survive.

Sunday   *Day 119*

Virginia is a twenty-seven-year-old woman having her first baby. She and her husband wrote a four-page letter to the hospital describing what they wanted by way of a birth experience: no drugs, no episiotomy, Jack's right to be with her at all times. When the letter arrived two weeks ago, staff were really angry, and one nurse even said, "She'd better not come in when I'm on, because I'm not about to take care of her."

Virginia came in early this morning and her labor had been following Hill's curve until she began pushing, and then her progress slowed down. When I walked into her room she was in a panic and said to me, "I might not make it." Her husband was there beside her, and also her cousin, who talked later of my calming influence on them all.

"Of course you'll make it," I told her, "but that's a common feeling." Half jokingly I added, "Anyway, you don't have much alternative."

"But it hurts so," she said between gritted teeth as a contraction ended.

"I know it does, but you know, you will survive."

"But what if I can't? What if I can't push the baby out?" I could see the panic in her eyes, the tension in her face, the white knuckles of her clenched fists as she asked the question.

"The bottom line is always the Caesarean."

She nodded with apparent relief. Her husband turned to me and snapped, "She's not ready for that yet," and I found myself angry at what seemed like insensitivity to his wife's pain.

"What about forceps?" she asked, searching for relief and an ending.

"That's been discussed, but you're not far along enough yet. It's still too soon."

The labor and her pushing went on and she delivered a beautiful baby, who breathed and cried and had perfect scores on the Apgar assessment.

I felt I had helped her have a vaginal delivery, that I had added to her strength. She was much more frightened than I had expected from her letter, which may have been motivated by fear more than strength.

I keep thinking about my upcoming meeting with Dr. Pierce. It is possible that he wants to see me about a patient I saw on rounds Friday whom I helped find an excuse for staying in the hospital. I'd found her in tears, saying that her baby was jaundiced but that she was being discharged anyway because we only allowed three days' hospitalization for an uncomplicated delivery. I suggested she develop "nausea," which would be a reason to keep her for observation another day but wouldn't require any immediate tests to be done on her. Her attending was furious with me when he found out and called Dr. Ingle, a close friend of Dr. Pierce's and also head of the Utilization Review Committee. Over the weekend Dr. Ingle wrote a letter authorizing the woman to stay.

Heather has an amazing ability when shopping to know exactly
what she wants for whom. I envy her lack of indecision. She
picked out a beautiful robe for me, and then she and I chose a
pair of pants for her. We then pretended we couldn't remember
what we had gotten for each other. The presents are all wrapped
under the tree, ready for a Christmas of just Heather and me.

Last night she fell asleep in my bed as I was sitting and
reading the newspaper. This morning she woke up at five as I
was having my morning coffee and reading the paper before
getting dressed. She thought it was still night and that I was still
reading the paper, so she couldn't understand why I was getting
up to get dressed.

"Mommy, do you like your job?" she asked.

"Well, there's a lot about it I don't like, but I do like taking
care of people and delivering babies."

"I wish you still worked in New Jersey because there it didn't
matter what time you got there or whether you came in."

That wasn't quite the reality of the job, but I was happy that
she perceived it that way.

Today is my meeting with Pierce.

Later

"Michelle, your charting is terrible. You haven't learned the
basic building blocks of obstetrics, the labor curve."

Feeling his anger sweeping over me, I made a weak response
—"I think that's a result of my general unhappiness with what
I see"—and then I began to weep. I had been caught and knew
I couldn't tell him the truth. The truth is that I have been
procrastinating in charting, because as soon as a woman's labor
is slightly different from the official labor curve, she is subjected
to treatment that may, in fact, make her worse. I haven't been
charting properly because I have been protecting women when
I could. In my confrontation with Dr. Pierce, I understood that

I had to play the game their way or get out. But I also know that every time I begin to plot a woman's labor curve, I feel that I am signing a death warrant. Sometimes I imagine I'm a guard at a concentration camp, admitting unsuspecting women who, if they do not behave according to the rules, will be sent to the gas chambers.

I was able to tell Pierce how unhappy I was about the amount of intervention, to which he responded, "Someday I'll tell you how hard it was when I was a resident." I found the remark irrelevant.

"It's worse at Memorial Hospital," he told me. "I don't know if you understand, Michelle, that you're training in a hospital known all over the world for its humaneness to patients as well as its effective technology."

"That's part of what's so hard to take," I replied. "If I were at Memorial, which is known to be different, known in obstetrics for its higher rate of intervention, I could think, 'At least it's better at Doctors, which is known for its policy of natural childbirth and nonintervention.'"

"Michelle, here you're studying with the best there are. We help set the standards for the rest of the country, if not the world, and they're good standards."

Pierce was by now being kindly and sympathetic as he suggested that I try harder with my charting.

Tuesday   *Day 120*

I would love to see the data on the incidence of Caesarean sections among those low-risk women approved for the Alternative Birth Service, because I suspect it is quite high. One of the attendings says that ABS really stands for "A Beautiful Section." The general rate in this hospital is one in five of those women who have not had a section before, and one in three of all women giving birth here. I do not believe this high rate is related to babies or mothers at risk. I remember a medical student last year who told me he would have to "hustle for sections" when he was a resident in OB-GYN. Here the residents don't have to hustle for sections; we just define a broad category of women who need them. My favorite indication is "maternal exhaustion." My friend Fran says that's when the doctor can't take any more. Last week a section was done because, according to the doctor, "She just couldn't take labor." Another chart recently read: "X-rays show room in pelvis. Will section to avoid trauma to baby."

Karen Dole challenged me at work today with, "How do you know that two hours isn't too much pushing?"

I answered, "How do you know that five minutes isn't too much?" then: "How do you know that a Caesarean is safe?"

A New York *Times* article on January 4, 1977, described the high rate (60 percent) of Caesareans in Brazil among women delivering in private clinics: " 'A substantial number of physicians in Brazil believe that the surgical delivery is the best method of childbirth—it causes no harm to the figure, it is quick, and it is a lot more profitable,' said Dr. Paolo Belfort de Aguiar, the former president of the Brazilian Federation of Gynecology and Obstetrics Associations."

The article went on to describe a woman who chose a Caesarean delivery "because 'some friends warned me' that a normal childbirth would somehow 'leave me internally deformed as far as sexual activity.' "

It is common practice after an episiotomy repair for the obstetrician to check the tightness of the woman's vagina and then announce she is "good as new."

A woman who has had a Caesarean instead of a vaginal delivery has an almost "perfect" vagina by such definitions. Never stretched by a baby's head, the vagina maintains its almost virginal state. In the Caesarean section, even the hymenal remnants, which are cut and then resewn during an episiotomy, are untouched.

No one at work thinks as I do. It's as though they have defined normal childbirth as the Caesarean section, and that vaginal delivery is appropriate only when there are special indications. I have fantasies in which women stand up in the thousands and thousands and say they are going to deliver their babies without having them cut out of their bellies.

Talking this afternoon with Nat Andrews at the School of Public Health helped me clarify why I am at the hospital and how long I ought to stay. He pointed out that getting my boards in OB-GYN wouldn't help me because I wouldn't be listened to, anyway. I told him I had given up my fantasies of rising through the ranks of the American College of Obstetrics and Gynecology and then being able to speak from a stronger position. I'd have to stay here another four years, then I'd have to practice in acceptable ways and not offend anyone in order to get my board certification. I realized that what they at the hospital define as the cure—i.e., the technology and surgery for childbirth—is what I define as the disease.

There is a comaraderie among physicians out of the mainstream, which includes public health physicians. Nat has invited Heather and me to have dinner with his family on Christmas Eve.

Thursday   *Day 123*

Heather ran a fever yesterday and complained of sore throat, headache and stiff neck. Worried about meningitis, I took her to see Catherine, my physician friend, who thought it was a strep throat. When we got home I collapsed in bed with Heather and felt sure I would never again have the strength to move. I put the TV where she could reach it and dozed on and off.

When I made the decision to stay home yesterday I didn't care if I was fired, but I felt that I was once again proving the validity of "Don't hire a woman. She'll stay home if her kid is sick." It is true, though, of me and other mothers, that we bring less to our work in terms of time and resources than people who aren't primarily responsible for children. I feel that what I am trying to do may not be possible. Louise is leaving tomorrow. Starting in ten days, I have night call again.

Later

Heather is much better today. She still has a belly ache and sore throat, but her fever is down and she's just a grumpy kid who isn't feeling well. I made it through!

Thursday morning (a week later)   *Day 130*

The past three days have been some of the most peaceful of my life. Heather, who slept until eleven on Christmas morning, has been in a lovely mood, giving our time together the quality it had when she was very little. I read, slept, wrote letters and puttered about the house while she played by herself and with friends. I spent several hours making tapes for friends in California and New Jersey. I hung the tape recorder around my neck and talked as I went about my day, chatting into the machine, pretending friends were here with me. When the tapes were done, I felt as though I'd been visiting.

I've been reading a fascinating book, *Woman and Nature,* by Susan Griffin, in which she describes most of our society as built around male constructs and male values. We do not recognize emotionality or intuition as basic components of our language or our truth. Her book supports my sense that at work they do not speak the same language I do. I find myself talking loudly, thinking that if I speak loud enough, they will hear me. The truth is that it is a different language altogether. For sixty hours a week now I live in a world in which I do not trust or believe in what I am doing, and where I have grave doubts about what I am inflicting on other human beings. It was so nice not to be there for three days.

On the way home

A thirty-year-old Mexican woman came into the hospital four weeks ago with a placenta previa. She was admitted for bed rest until she is closer to term, when she would be sectioned. The woman, who spoke no English, had other children at home, including a one-year-old, and she signed herself out without permission several times. The psychiatrist said she was disturbed, largely because of her determination to be home with the others. She was on John's floor, so I had no direct contact with her, but from a distance, I was never sure she understood why she was here. She was a small thin woman who was sometimes seen wandering in the hall, looking depressed, confused and alone. Today they took her in for the section. Something went wrong and there was massive hemorrhaging. Additional teams of both doctors and nurses were called in, and when I left they were taking out her uterus altogether in an attempt to stop the bleeding.

Left alone to watch L&D, I admitted an eighteen-year-old who was having her first baby. She was accompanied by her sister, who, when she saw me, asked, "Who are you, anyway?" It was like the day I met Nancy Carr and we recognized something in each other. It is like the language about which Susan Griffin writes and the unspoken signals that communicate understanding.

I answered softly to her, "I'm the resident and I'll tell you the rest later." Then I checked Janet, her sister.

The girl's cervix was almost fully dilated and the baby's head almost out. Since she was a midwife service patient, I called Susan, who was going on duty shortly, and she said she would come up. Although Janet didn't want an episiotomy, I told her I might have to do one because I was afraid the midwife's attending might show up and be critical of my not doing one. When Susan arrived I was holding the episiotomy scissors. I turned to her, and knowing that she often did episiotomies, said, "I think there might not be enough room, so I'll have to do an episiotomy." She nodded in agreement.

However, I let Janet keep her legs together between contractions and I let the drapes fall over her legs so no one else knew that the baby's head was almost out. I did perineal massage with sterile ointment on my fingers, and under the drapes was able to slowly let the perineal tissue stretch, more slowly than anyone would have allowed me to do. All the time I held the scissors, pretending that I was about to do the episiotomy. The baby was born during one of the contractions and I said, "Oops, too late for the episiotomy."

After the delivery I talked with Diana, Janet's sister from New Jersey, who wants to be a midwife, and knows one of the babies I delivered at home. Diana was happy I was there, but she'd expected me to be there, or someone like me. She had dreamed about the delivery, so she expected that it would go exactly as it did.

Although Janet had no tears I could find, I kept having the feeling that maybe she was so torn that what I thought was intact perineum must have been a tear through her rectum. They have me so brainwashed that I can't even believe my own eyes when I see an intact perineum.

I had to leave because Heather was due to be dropped off at the house after being taken skating. I drove away from the hospital, already having stayed an hour late, with mixed feelings about Janet's delivery and the tear I worried I'd missed, and about the surgery I was missing.

I arrived home to find that Maggie had had diarrhea all over the dining-room floor. I cleaned it up, then washed the floor and swept the rest of the downstairs. On my knees scrubbing, feeling angry, I thought, They think all I want to do is go home and take it easy. They don't know I go home to clean up the dog shit.

Friday   *Day 131*

I went back and checked Janet this morning, and of course she has no tears at all.

Irv Warren likes to challenge me, I think. This morning, scrubbing at the sinks before a delivery, he asked, "You don't approve of what I'm doing, do you?"

He's right. I don't. He had been screaming at the woman in the delivery room, yelling "Push! Push!," then, "You lazy female, push!" When she whimpered, "I'm trying," he yelled, "You're not trying hard enough. Now push!" and his large round face became red and his belly puffed out, making him a fearsome figure.

At the sinks I responded to his question, "Well, that's not how I would do it," and shrugged, trying not to show how strongly I felt.

He stopped scrubbing for a moment and in a patronizing way said, "Michelle, when people are in a subservient position, sometimes you just have to tell them what to do."

Implicit in obstetrics is the presumption that women having babies are subservient to their doctors. My own giving birth was no different. My due date had been November 30. Passing me in the hospital corridor on that date, Andy, my obstetrician and colleague said, "Michelle, today is your due date. Why don't you let me induce you? Aren't you tired of waiting?"

"Can't let you induce me, Andy. You'll mess up the kid's sun signs."

My being a physician made Andy nervous. Taking care of colleagues is always difficult. "If anything is going to go wrong, it will happen with you," he had told me.

Two days later, on Saturday morning, I went into labor. Making rounds that morning, I had to stop every fifteen or twenty minutes to rest until the contraction passed. I felt my body about to erupt, but I needed to keep going. For most of my life, school and then work had been the stabilizing forces and I was afraid to stop.

Eventually I lay down on my bed. Then I felt a flood of warm water seeping out of my vagina, soaking me and my bed.

I called Ellen, the friend who was going to coach me through labor. She was the only woman I knew in town who had had natural childbirth and was breast-feeding. "My membranes have ruptured," I told her.

"That's wonderful. Don't you want to go in?"

"No, I'm fine here for a while."

"I need to put Susie down for a nap, but I'll stop by for a short visit first."

Soon Ellen arrived with her girl. Susie, a lively but gentle toddler, climbed up on the bed and patted my belly as she had been doing for some months. Then she stretched out on top of me and I enjoyed the presence of the two babies together, one still inside and the other draped over my pregnant abdomen.

Ellen left and I began to think about what I knew of ruptured membranes. What if the baby's head was still high? (I knew this wasn't so, because I had checked myself.) I was still filled with "What if's?" This was me, not a patient, and I couldn't remember what was serious and what I could ignore. I was a woman having contractions, caught up in my body's process, and vulnerable.

Once in the hospital, I was placed flat in bed and told not to move except onto my side. I stared at the bare pale-green walls. Ellen arrived, and dismayed by the starkness, hung on the wall a tie she was sewing for her husband. For the rest of the afternoon and evening I lay staring at the psychedelic red-and-orange tie, holding Ellen's hand through the raised siderails of the bed.

At ten o'clock at night Andy told me I had another eight hours to go. The thought of that much time left must have further stimulated my labor because by eleven he was getting ready to take me to the delivery room. Ellen, who had been so much a part of the labor, was left at the door. She said later she understood how fathers feel being left behind.

Moved onto the table, I protested, "No, I don't want my hands strapped." But my arms were strapped to the table. My legs were put into the stirrups and suddenly I was trapped, both by the forces within my body and by the people around me.

Episiotomy? In my sixth month I had told Andy I didn't want one. "But you have to," he had insisted. "It's for your own good. You'll get loose and that won't be very pleasurable for a man in intercourse."

"It doesn't seem to have hurt anyone for all the centuries women didn't have episiotomies. They keep having babies, so they must be having intercourse."

He said, "That's only because no man ever turns anything down."

Now, three months later, strapped to the delivery table, I told him, "I'm not going to tie your hands for this delivery. You have to do it the way you know how."

There was a lot of bustle as the table was tilted back. Andy's fingers were in my vagina and then he told me, "The kid has hair and I can see it." Reaching for the scissors, he said, "I'm going to do the episiotomy on the next contraction and then I'm going to tell you to push."

I felt my flesh being cut, creating a searing pain which at that moment didn't seem to matter.

"Push," he said, and I felt released from within me a force and direction I had been practicing for as long as I could remember. My baby flew out and suddenly there was a commotion.

"I didn't tell you to push that hard!" Andy shrieked. "Look what you've done!"

I thought, Why is this man screaming at me? I've just had a baby.

"You have a healthy girl here, but dammit, why did you have to push so hard?"

My baby was put in my arms for a moment, then whisked away. I wanted her back. I wanted to see her, hold her, celebrate her, celebrate that I had pushed her out of my body.

Andy had done the episiotomy and then, breaking an important first rule, had looked away as he put the scissors back onto the table behind him. In the second he wasn't looking, my baby had come flying out and landed in his lap. Because there was no control of the birth, the episiotomy had extended down through my rectum.

"This is going to take a lot of sewing," he said, now calmed down and somewhat apologetic.

"It's okay," I told him. I wasn't afraid of anything now. My baby was alive and crying. I just wanted it to be over. The stitches hurt as Andy sewed together the parts of my anal sphincter, my rectum, and my vagina.

There was a party in my room with Ellen, her husband and some other friends. Andy had brought champagne so we could celebrate. Then, at two in the morning, they brought my baby to me. I lay there and stared and wondered about our life together. I studied what she looked like and by morning she looked like what my baby should look like.

I spent a wonderful day out in the country meeting with some women on a project that will look at the effects of culture on biology, instead of biology on culture. I think how many women are having Caesarean sections and how their children will think that is the way babies are born. The culture will have changed.

The weather was beautiful, giving me a wonderful sense of freedom as we drove south along the lake.

Murray Avery, a young obstetrician interested in both natural childbirth and monitors, spoke to me yesterday about a study he wants to do on anxiety in labor. I tried to explain that we do not have the right language for the feelings that may be affecting labor. All his study can show is the relationship of the course of labor to a defined scale of "one to ten" of levels of anxiety. This may all be irrelevant to what we are actually experiencing in labor. He wants to quantify our experiences.

"My wife is having contractions and now she wants to push." A husband was on the phone to the OB unit, and I said to bring her in right away, now.

They arrived about fifteen minutes later. Vilma, black, twenty-eight, was having her second baby, her husband was with her. They were both doing breathing exercises well and obviously in control. Vilma's cervix was eight centimeters dilated, and I sensed she was going to deliver quickly. I called the midwife who was covering, and also the attending who backs up the midwives.

Rachel, the nurse watching Vilma, asked me to check her again quickly because she thought the baby was coming soon. This time Vilma was fully dilated and her bag of waters, the membranes, were still intact. As Vilma pushed, the bag of waters would bulge out and actually stretch the perineum.

"What's that?" Rachel asked with an expression of dismay.

"Those are the membranes stretching the perineum."

"I've never seen a delivery where the membranes haven't been ruptured. It looks so strange." Rachel had been there two years.

"The membranes and the water help stretch the perineum before the baby's head gets there and the fluid helps protect the baby."

Vilma delivered slowly, pushing gently, with no episiotomy. The baby cried and then quickly settled down in her mother's arms.

The attending arrived right after the baby was born, and the midwife half an hour later.

Monday   Day 134

This last day on OB was fourteen hours long, spent primarily with Jackie, my chief, and Hilda Cameron, the attending for the majority of women in labor throughout the day. Jackie, Hilda and I spent much of this fourteen-hour day talking.

During the day Esther, a seventeen-year-old Puerto Rican, tall and massively obese, arrived on the floor. She said, "I'm here to have my baby today. My baby was due last week and I want it now."

She'd had no recent prenatal care, and didn't plan to return after today. She was adamant that she would have her baby today and that we were to make it happen. After asking her some questions, I tried to examine her, but she was terrified and would not let me touch her. I said I had to examine her, and the nurse backed me up. When Esther let herself be uncovered, I could see huge warts covering her labia, so it was difficult even to find her vaginal opening. As I tried to insert the speculum she pulled her whole body away from me, up toward the head of the bed. When I tried to reach her, she pulled farther away, her eyes bulging. She looked like a cornered caged animal, and I stopped.

I called Jackie, who I knew would want to examine her anyway, so my exam would have been superfluous. I also expected

Jackie to do better than I because people, like veins, sometimes know who has more authority and respond differently.

When Jackie tried to examine the girl, however, she had no more success. Esther, still terrified, pulled back, drew her legs together, and would not let herself be touched. Jackie was obviously getting angry, and after two tries, ripped off her gloves and left the room. Once outside, she turned to me and to the nurse and said, "Women like that prove that no woman can be raped unless she wants to."

Realizing how shocked the nurse and I were, she qualified that by saying, "Well, maybe with a gun or a knife . . ." Jackie calls herself a feminist. She is known as a feminist physician. Women will come to her because they believe she is different from men.

I wanted especially to do well with Hilda today, since she was the attending with me on my first day on OB. Today I delivered a patient of hers with an episiotomy, then did the repair as Hilda wanted it. She complimented me on my skills and then went on to tease me about my trouble doing an episiotomy the first day.

Hilda shared with me some of her life, saying she found it easier to talk with women who had children. When she has two hours free, she runs home to do things no one else will do. She straightens up her house because her sitter will quit if the house is too messy and because "I have to keep my house neat or I'll lose my husband."

Jackie joined us for a while and Hilda asked if Jackie has children.

"No, but I probably will. My husband wants them."

"Well," Hilda said in a resigned way, "most women have children for their husbands, anyway."

Pity for them came over me. I always wanted a child more than I wanted a husband. I imagine having children for someone else must be terrible, and not any fun.

I have finally mastered running the pH analyzer as well as calibrating it for accuracy, something I've been working on for a while in spite of Richard's insistence that I didn't need to know how, since he could run all the samples.

Hilda had a woman in labor today who had a questionable monitor tracing, so she tried to get a pH sample. The woman was in heavy labor and kept moving onto her side, trying to find a more comfortable position, but Hilda had to keep moving her onto her back. Using the disposable pH kit, Hilda took the long tube, shaped like a megaphone and about eight inches long, and inserted the narrower end into the woman's vagina. She tried to get it through the slightly dilated cervix, which was especially difficult because the woman moved a lot whenever she had a contraction.

Hilda was unable twice to get the tube set right on the baby's head. After her second attempt she handed the tube to me while she got ready to do it for a third time. When Jackie happened to walk into the room, Hilda turned to her and asked if she would try. As Jackie opened a new kit and got ready to try, she said to me, "Michelle, the reason you had so much trouble getting a sample . . . ," thinking because I was holding the tube, I was the one that had failed. Hilda did not set her straight.

It wasn't until the day was over that I realized it had been a day spent mostly with women doctors, and yet it had been no different from other days at the hospital.

Last year, teaching at the medical school, I was on a panel about women's health. I was asked by an angry obstetrician, "Are you trying to say that OB-GYN should only be practiced by women?"

"No, I'm not saying that," I responded, much to his surprise, "because the women in the field are not unlike the men. The problem is with some of the basic practices and basic assumptions about women that are an integral part of the profession. The same system, with women replacing the men, would not change it significantly."

Although I said those words, I had not been without some hope that it really would be different if the doctors were women.

Chapter Ten

Beep, beep. My pager calls me, catches me, ties me like a long umbilical cord to the hospital switchboard and anyone who calls. I'm free, though, of L&D, of Richard as my chief, of asking permission to leave the floor. I can even fantasize turning off my beeper and being unreachable, saying later, "There must have been something wrong with my beeper."

Returning to GYN also gives me back the on-call room, a converted patient room with two beds, a desk, some lockers, and a closet for coats. It is a room only for women, so occasionally there is even a spirit of friendliness in there. It is a room with a telephone, where I can call home, make contact with the rest of my life.

Jackie is my chief; Thomas, someone I don't know very well, is the third-year resident; Karen Dole and I share the second-year position; and John is the first-year resident. Barbara and Richard are only peripherally part of the team, as they are on the abortion and outpatient service. However, since both of them refuse to do abortions, the rest of us do the procedures on their patients, while they do the work-ups and follow-up care.

Jackie and I were in the OR from eight to noon, doing one D&C, which probably wasn't necessary, and two abortions, which could have been done elsewhere more cheaply and with less depersonalization. The OR costs $350 an hour—for the room alone. That's $1,400 for the three procedures this morning.

Back on the GYN floor at one, I began the work-ups for the afternoon. The medical history includes the question of occupation, so I asked Mrs. Ack, "Are you employed outside the home?"

"No. I have a college education—do you have any suggestions?"

Mrs. Ack was the wife of a VIP, admitted for a procedure she didn't need. We had established an instant rapport, which made this work-up pleasurable.

"I don't have any special ideas. Are you looking for something?" I said as I went about examining her.

"I've spent twenty-five years as a housewife and mother—and that counts for nothing on my résumé," she responded. Then, after some moments of silence, she added, "I've done twenty-five years of volunteer work, but it counts for nothing because I wasn't paid."

There was a knock on the door and then Richard's voice saying he needed the room. Feeling free of his power over me, I asked, "Need a pelvic, dear?"

"Just don't take too long, Michelle, I need the room."

I turned to Mrs. Ack and said, "He used to be my chief and I had to listen to him, but he isn't anymore."

We went on talking about women and work. There was the closeness between us that unites all women. In health care the abuses of women cut across all classes, with unneeded surgery for the "privileged" and neglect for the underprivileged.

Later as I passed the treatment room I could see John examining a woman. The curtain had been only partly pulled across the room, so although she was covered with a sheet, through the window I could see John's head and face, and the sheet over the woman's knees. It was a framed and eerie picture—a vain and handsome man looking into the bottom half of a woman, who had no identity.

Heather says her stomach hurts when she sits at her desk. She is far behind the others in her class, but when I speak with her about repeating first grade she cries and says she wants to go on with her friends. I know she will survive but I keep thinking about how she's had to sacrifice for my being in this program.

Fran and Laurie seem to think I made some errors in hiring baby-sitters the last few times, so they are going to advertise and screen applicants. They seem to believe there is a right person to hire. In the meantime they are once again taking turns staying at the house to see Heather off in the morning, and they are filling in for the four hours a week between sitters.

Later

Jackie seems amazed at how easily we get along. She keeps expecting me to give her trouble, but I have been totally accepting of her decisions and of her power to make them. Yesterday I saw the OR schedule and asked Jackie if I could scrub on a hysterectomy with Dr. MacDougal, who gave me a lot of surgery on OB. "But Thomas has higher rank than you do, Michelle, so I have to give him first choice." She has apparently decided to give me the case, though, leaving me wondering what price I shall have to pay for that favor.

Thursday   *Day 137*

"A twelve-week-size uterus is about the size of a grapefruit," I was telling Caroline, the medical student also scrubbed in on the hysterectomy with Dr. MacDougal. He was teaching me as we did the hysterectomy, and I was passing on what I knew to the medical student. This woman had a fibroid tumor which had enlarged her uterus to the size of a twelve-week pregnancy. The three of us were busily working at tying off vessels, probing, chatting, when Dr. MacDougal, holding one ovary gently in his hand, showed us a small cyst on the surface and said, "I just might take it out. She doesn't need two."

Suddenly worried that this woman's ovary was being so easily discarded, I tried an oblique way to argue for its being left in place. "Dr. MacDougal, I've heard of women having hormonal problems after a hysterectomy even when both ovaries are left in. What causes that?"

"I don't really know, Michelle, but it happens. I personally think that even if we are careful there is still a cutting off of some of the blood supply to the ovaries when we take out the uterus. They just don't always work as well as before."

Glancing at Caroline, hoping she understood what I was trying to do, I said to MacDougal, "But if it's possible that this surgery will hurt her ovary, then if we take one out, she is more vulnerable to any damage done to the one left in."

Just then Johnson, the fertility expert, walked in and said, "Mac?"

"Yeah," Dr. MacDougal answered. "Hi there. What's up?"

"I was just wondering if you were planning to take out any ovaries this morning. I need some for culture."

"Well, I was thinking about it. Let me think about it some more," he said and turned to me. "You know they don't work as well after hysterectomy."

"Yes, but if you take the one with the cyst, she might end up with none working."

"Maybe you're right."

"She's only thirty-two, and I think she still wants them," I added.

Johnson shrugged and said, "I don't want to push you. I was just asking," and left.

Later Caroline and I overheard Johnson talking with Enders out in the hall. "I see you have a hysterectomy later today. Are you taking out the ovaries on her?"

"Well, I hadn't made up my mind yet, John. Why?"

"I'm looking for ovaries. I need some."

"Well, I guess I could." Enders paused as though to say more.

"Don't do it for my sake," Johnson interjected, but he had his arm on Enders' shoulder, their closeness making evident the danger to Enders' patient's ovaries.

As Caroline and I walked away, I said to her, "They sure don't do that with testicles."

Yesterday I admitted a woman as an infertility case, but when I discovered it was her husband who was sterile, I found myself reluctant to put on the chart a description of his infertility. I suddenly realized the sexism of my own attitude. We label women infertile all the time, yet even I find myself reluctant to so label a man for fear of what it will do to him and for fear of how others will respond to him. We protect testicles and take out ovaries.

Later

Mel Diamond, a physician who attends homebirths in Everytown called me three weeks ago and said, "I've heard you are having trouble at the hospital. I'd like to help if I can."

We arranged to meet at my house tonight, and then I thanked him for his offer. I had called Mel last year to offer my support when I heard he was attending home births and I knew that he was now trying to work out an agreement with Pierce for backup care of home-birth patients who might need hospitalization.

Within minutes after he arrived tonight, he said with surprise, "Oh! I thought your problems were personal. What you're telling me is that things are bad at the hospital."

"Mel, you ought to know. Look what happened to the two women you brought in."

Shortly before I left OB, Mel's partner had brought in a woman with a breech baby for vaginal delivery. She was sent for x-rays to check the exact position of the baby, but by the time she came back, she had almost delivered. As she was being taken into the delivery room someone glanced at the x-ray and said that the head was at the wrong angle for a vaginal delivery, that it was deflexed, in a poor position. The films, however, were never carefully examined. Because the baby was almost out, the woman was rushed to the section table. The anesthesiologist, failing to get the spinal needle in place, tried to give the woman general anesthesia. She began to scream for them to stop because she didn't want it. She was held down and put to sleep. The baby, delivered by section, was tiny, had congenital abnormalities incompatible with life, and died shortly after birth.

The next day I argued with a nurse about the delivery. "You know, we had no right to put her under if she was refusing anesthesia."

"But she had to have the operation for the sake of the baby," the nurse argued.

"But that's her decision. It's her body being cut into."

"No! She has no right to make that decision, and even if she refused a section, we had the right to operate." The nurse glared angrily at me, giving me the sense I had just been classified among child murderers because I thought a woman had the right to decide if her belly was going to be cut open.

Mel knew the story but had never heard it from this perspective. Silent for a moment, he said, "It's as though we only concentrate on the baby and not on the mother at all. I wonder why that is." I didn't know how to answer that question for him.

As we talked more about breech babies Mel mentioned the 20 percent chance of spinal injury if the head is deflexed.

"Mel, I think everyone is having a deflexed head these days. They are either very deflexed, a little deflexed or minimally deflexed. But, somehow, I doubt that suddenly all the heads on babies have changed."

Mel looked thoughtfully at me, so I went on, "You practiced in rural Canada for years and delivered a lot of breeches. How many spinal injuries did you see?"

He shook his head and said, "None." Then he added, "But you know, Michelle, I feel good about the OBs who've said they are willing to back me up and take care of my emergencies. It's not altogether bad there. They're trying to make progress."

"Well, I see it from the inside. What you get from that group is not support, but a lack of concern about who does what with their patients."

Friday *Day 138*

It was beautiful to be able to take Heather to school in the morning and to meet her at three when she got out. I brought Maggie with me to meet her and to walk home with us. Heather, in her clogs, ran across the hill with Maggie barking and running. I love to see them together. Heather's hair is the color of Maggie's Sheltie coat. When they lie next to each other, their hair is almost indistinguishable. Heather teases me about the time they were both on my bed and I was saying "Nice Maggie" as I stroked what I thought was the dog's hair.

It's four o'clock now and I'm heading into work for the next seventeen hours, dreading how I will feel at the end of that time. It's like taking Ipecac to make you throw up and knowing how miserable you're going to be when it takes effect. It's like walking out in the cold without a jacket and knowing you're going to be freezing. It's doing violence to myself and I don't know how long I can do that.

Tuesday *Day 142*

One of the applicants for the job of baby-sitter sounded so wonderful on the phone that Fran and Laurie wanted me to see her right away. Last night she came to the house and told us her last job was as a sex-therapy surrogate, which she finally decided was prostitution. She is applying for Social Security Disability because she is chronically ill. She cannot tolerate either heat or stress. In the hour she was with us she never said hello or anything else to Heather.

This morning I woke to a flooded basement, so I went out and chopped a trench to let the water run off from the downspout, which was sending it into the cellar. Last fall I tried several times to get someone out to fix the gutters because I knew this would happen eventually.

On the way home

Jackie and I were at the sinks scrubbing before our first case when she said, "Oh, this is Tuesday, the day you are off in the afternoon."

"No, don't you remember? I gave up my afternoon time off to be able to leave at five-thirty instead of six."

"How long is this going to last?" she asked in a sulky way.

"I don't know. Yesterday we interviewed someone terrible. I'm trying the best I can."

Jackie scrubbed the brush against her hand harder and harder, leaving red streaks from the bristles. I could see and feel her anger. Pausing in her scrubbing, she glared at me and said, "You don't realize how psychologically devastating it is when you leave at five-thirty."

"There's not much I can do about that," I said. "After four months it seems that whatever I do is psychologically devastating. I'm trying to respond to my own sense of fairness. I've given up trying to please you."

We both noticed the anesthesiologist waving frantically because the patient was already asleep on the table. We went into the operating room, and with discussion restricted to technical detail only, did an abortion. Once the case was over, we went out and talked some more.

"I've been surprised at how little responsibility you take, Michelle. It really surprises me."

"What are you talking about?"

"You should be doing pelvic exams in the holding area to see if abortion patients are having the right procedure."

"Isn't that a bit late, Jackie? Isn't that why Barbara and Richard see them and schedule them? If they can't check them accurately, then they are the problem." I thought about what the holding area was like, one large room full of stretchers with curtains between them which often didn't even close all the way. It didn't seem the right time to be asking someone why or when or how they got pregnant and then checking to see how large the uterus is.

"I just think you should be more interested and more involved." I felt like a naughty child being scolded. "You should have more of a personal sense of responsibility."

She was touching on the core of my compromise in being here. "Being personally responsible, though, implies some influence over what will be done. I have come to accept that I will learn procedures, but I have little say in what happens to any patient."

"But you have to be responsible for what you do," she told me in a strident voice.

Anger and tears which she may not have noticed welled up, and with a trembling voice I told her, "I can't accept responsibility for anything I've done in the past three months of obstetrics. I did what I was told to do. How can I feel personally responsible when my opinion is meaningless?"

I feel terrible about what I said, for I really know that I am personally responsible and it is a denial of that truth which allows me to be here. Deep down I know I am responsible for my actions, even when under orders.

Jackie and I ended our discussion with her saying, "It must be terrible to be doing things for which you wouldn't want to feel responsible."

A terrible sore has appeared on my wrist, a long stinging straight line, as though I had been burned. It is red and oozes fluid. Its presence on my body is so strange. I've no memory of how I got it. It seems to have come from inside, where the pain of this job resides.

Wednesday   *Day 143*

The anterior-posterior (A-P) repair is basically a tightening of the upper and lower portions of the vagina. It gives more support to the bladder and urethra as well as to the rectum. At the same time, it makes the vaginal opening smaller. Dr. Core,

Thomas and I did a hysterectomy and then A-P repair on a woman who was having this procedure done partly because her husband was impotent. The husband's psychiatrist had called Dr. Core to suggest to her that the woman's loose vagina was contributing to her husband's impotence and the procedure might help him. We were standing, all three of us, squeezed between the woman's stirruped legs, measuring the opening of her vagina, wondering how tight to make it, when I said jokingly, "Maybe her husband should have been told his penis was too small, not that her vagina was too loose."

Everyone was laughing as we continued taking turns putting two fingers into the woman's vagina, trying to guess the right size, when I suggested, "I think the husband ought to have been measured, then we could get a dildo of the right size and tighten the vagina around the dildo to make it the correct size." They were all enjoying my humor, oblivious of my rage at this woman's vagina being fashioned to fit her impotent husband.

This morning at Grand Rounds, Cassie Connor gave an eloquent and moving talk on pain control and the psychological approaches to cancer patients. The trouble is that she never does any of the things she spoke of or recommended; instead she leaves us to cover for the patients from whom she withdraws when they are in pain and dying.

Thursday   *Day 144*

I received a call last night from the chairman of the department of family medicine at a medical school, offering me the directorship of a new residency program. I told him I was planning to stay on here and get more training.

Bill, one of the first-year residents, has left the program, although no one seems sure why.

Everyone is in an uproar and worried about how to cover the OB service with one person less. There is a possibility I might be moved to night OB. At a residents meeting today everyone was fighting with everyone else over who had more work to do.

The chief residents, who used to tell us how terrible the first years were, complained that the residents now have it too easy.

Friday   Day 145

The system in which I am functioning now has so many stress points, I worry about something going wrong.

I'm not sure if I can make it here but I will be very depressed if I have to quit. Maybe I never should have tried, but now that I am here, I do not want to leave. Certainly, without help I can't go on. This evening Fran and Laurie are coming with Bea, a candidate for the job. I need someone badly.

Dr. Pierce has hired a new resident to start in two weeks, so that crisis in the program is over.

The conization of the cervix is an operation in which the inside of the cervix is cut out, similar to the way an apple is cored in the center, but with a wider amount being cut off the outside than the inside. It is a bloody, deforming procedure which I learned to do today. It is done to remove areas of cancerous tissue or other abnormal cells.

During laparoscopy today, I found myself staring at the tubes coming out of the woman's belly and vagina, wondering if the women would be so willing to have the surgery if they knew what was being done to them. No one should be asleep for surgery.

Saturday   Day 146

Bea came to dinner Friday night. She is a slight, pale woman in her late twenties, who is trying to decide what to do with her life. She was intrigued by Fran's ad, which described the job in my house in quite glorious terms. In addition we discovered that she has worked in women's health clinics and has friends in common with Fran. We all liked her. She was friendly and spoke with Heather, who still looks so easily to the next person and asks, "Are you going to be my next baby-sitter?"

I'm missing the fun of mothering, but I see this time as tempo-rary. I find myself thinking about having another child and raising my children within a community of women. How rela-tionships with men and getting pregnant fit into that plan is unknown, but I feel a commonality with other women in terms of child raising that doesn't exist for me in relationships with men.

Two weeks have passed—one twenty-fifth of what is ahead this year—since I began marking off days on my year-at-a-glance calendar.

The road is icy and treacherous as I drive in for another thirty-six-hour shift. Last night, speaking to some pre-med stu-dents at a dinner, I realized that when I walk into the hospital, there is no one with whom I can talk.

School is closed tomorrow, leaving me in need of two full days of child care, so Heather is staying at Catherine's until tomor-row night.

Yesterday morning Larry Morris let me do most of a ruptured ovarian cyst after we did the laparoscopy and saw that the woman was bleeding internally. Larry encourages my aggres-siveness in doing what I can in surgery. He told me a story of when he was a resident and scrubbed with Bob Carter on a section. Bob wasn't letting Larry do enough, so Larry "acciden-tally" nicked one of Bob's gloves, which forced Bob to step out to change gloves while Larry delivered the baby. In doing the surgery, I was especially careful not to jeopardize the patient because of my inexperience, so I only did what I was certain I could manage.

Standing over the OR table with Larry, I realized that the next day we were scheduled to be back together in the OR doing another ovarian cyst, but in the interim he would go home for the day and night, while I had to go on working during all that time.

In the night I slept short periods of about an hour each, between trips to the ER to see women with problems often weeks old that suddenly seemed urgent. I remember once waking up after I had come back to the on-call room, suddenly thinking I had to go to the ER. I jumped out of bed, then remembered I had just been there, then couldn't remember if I had. I decided to go back to sleep, and that if it had been the ER calling, they'd call again.

People who come to the emergency room often have problems which have been present for days or weeks. On Sunday nights this is especially true when we see people who are lonely after a weekend alone, or unable to face the new week, or scared because they must be better by Monday morning. Sunday night is a crisis time in many people's lives, and in crisis, one's body becomes a reason to seek help, company, reassurance.

Today I was back in the OR with Larry, operating on another ovarian cyst. He said repeatedly, "Michelle, Dr. Pierce would be proud of how well you are doing, even if the rest of the surgery doesn't go well." I had been working carefully and diligently, trying to remove the cysts without their breaking. "You have excellent hands," he said, making me feel quite victorious. If I got fired today, I had proven I could do surgery. This operation was especially pleasurable because it was delicate work, no one was telling me to hurry, and Larry obviously respected my work. I told Jackie at sign-out, "I fought to keep every millimeter of her good ovarian tissue."

Tuesday morning   *Day 149*

An incredibly wonderful back rub by Catherine put me to sleep in front of her fireplace. Catherine has magic in her hands. They seem to exist not as physical objects but as a great warmth spreading over my back and neck. I slept until Heather woke me with "Are you awake, Mama?" It was not until ten that we got home and I finally settled Heather down in my bed.

I called Fran to ask about Bea's references, and then called Bea to say I wanted to hire her. Bea said she was looking forward to being Heather's "nanny." She said that they might have difficulties along the way but that Heather wasn't an angry child. I wasn't sure what she meant, but I thought she was making reference to what she thought of the children of working mothers. I can't say I'm convinced Bea is the "right person," but she has good references and I desperately need help: Fran and Laurie will leave for the East Coast; Gail will be away at school; and in two weeks I begin a long stretch of night call.

Heather had a beautiful time at Catherine's, so she was in good shape when I brought her home last night. It's all gone so well, and although I'm still tired and short of sleep, I feel optimistic.

Later

Gail tried to reach me all morning to say Heather was home sick, but the OR secretary wasn't letting the calls through. Heather sounded tired and down when I finally talked with her at two, but it's probably nothing more than her sore throat.

Larry and I again stood facing each other across the operating table on which a woman lay with a huge ovarian cyst, and I said to him, "Larry, we can't keep meeting this way." John had been scrubbed with him, but had suddenly developed a severe stomach ache and had to step out, so I was called in to replace him. When I arrived, the cyst had been brought out of the abdominal cavity and Larry was planning to clamp it and cut it off when I suggested that he let me do it the way I had done the last two: dissecting it out instead of cutting it off because I could then preserve more of the ovarian tissue. Larry agreed, allowing me to do the surgery with little bleeding and without breaking the cyst or removing any extra tissue. "Michelle, your hands are so good, why don't you go into infertility surgery?" was his comment today.

George Guin let me do a cone biopsy today, which surprised me because I haven't done a lot with him. There is a strange ritual dance taking place as it is being decided who will do a case, involving a balance between aggressive and nonaggressive behavior. The patient today had her legs up in stirrups, with both George and me standing between them when the nurse asked, "Will you be sitting or standing?" George said, "Yes, one of us will be sitting." The nurse lowered the table and put a stool there between the woman's legs but neither of us sat on it. I wouldn't presume he would let me do the case, yet neither did I move out of the way so he could sit down. We started to do the surgery with both of us leaning over and bending, since the patient had already been lowered. Finally he said to me, "Michelle, why don't you sit down?"—letting me know the case was mine.

Wednesday   Day 150

Dr. MacDougal and I were scrubbed on a mini-lap when he asked, "Have you done any?"

"No," I answered, knowing I probably could have bluffed through.

"I'll do this one, and you can do the next," he told me. Part way through, however, it was clear I knew what I was doing, so he let me take over. There is a subtleness to the exchange that implies, "Let me do this now. I know what I am doing."

Standing at the table doing the tubal ligation, I could see into the next operating room where I knew Dr. Johnson was doing a tubal re-anastamosis, or retying of tubes. I thought, It's like a supermarket. In one room a woman is having her tubes tied, and in the other a woman is having them sewn back together again. It could be an auto-body shop.

Thursday   Day 151

Today, doing abortions, scraping out the insides of women's uteri, I became clear that women and fetuses are victims in our society, pitted against one another, without options.

Doug Weston, who supervises the abortion service, is an aggressive young macho attending. As I was scrubbing the patient he told me to change the way I held the sponge stick. I asked, "What's the difference?" knowing I was being rebellious, but that there really is no difference. Then as I was taking the instruments out of the sterilizer, a job I was doing because we were short of nurses, I tried to put the instruments in the order in which I would be using them. Doug said, "Stop what you are doing. You must do it the way I tell you. Otherwise we have role reversal here."

I saw another side of Doug in the OR one day. He was doing an abortion and said, "Some people have accused me of being a baby-killer, but I'm doing what I think is right."

Tuesday   *Day 156*

Heather and I spent three beautiful days on High Island resting, reading, walking, playing. We were due back Sunday but storms closed the boatline, so we had to stay another night and day until the winds died down enough for the ferry to run. I miss being close to the ocean, which makes time at the lake even more special. Being near the water was soothing, leaving me feeling at one with the world.

The break from the hospital and the pressures of home made me wonder why I was doing this to myself. Standing on the sand, Heather searching and finding pebbles to put in a bag, I found myself questioning, "Why am I working as I am?" . . . "Why am I cutting up the bodies of women?" . . . "Why am I working with people whose values I detest, whose choices I do not respect?" Heather's voice saying, "Look at this shell, Mama," diverted me periodically from those thoughts. I didn't want to think that way, yet why was I going back? What was I going to do in the end? Did I really want what I had been fighting so hard to hold on to for the past five months?

We arrived home last night to find Bea moved in and settled before the fire. Seeing her gave me a sense of peace and calm;

I was rested and felt a strong hope that she would be the relief I needed. This is the stretch of time for which we all knew I would need help. As I left for work this morning I felt that the pieces were all in order.

Later

"Heather is an unmanageable and uncontrolled child!" Bea was on the phone yelling at me, having managed to get a call through to me in the OR.

My sense of well-being shattered, I wanted instantly to be home. "What happened?" I asked, trying to be calm, waiting for the story, frightened by the anger in Bea's voice.

"Heather came home at one and refused to eat the lunch I fixed her. She said she was going to her room to watch TV. I said she couldn't, so she started to cry and scream."

"Where is she now? Let me speak to her." I didn't understand.

"Heather, what happened?" I asked from a small desk in the supply area of the OR. Around me moved figures in green, masked and gowned, getting bottles off racks, hooking up tubing, searching for labels on sterilized instruments.

"Mama," Heather was crying, "I just wanted to go to my room to watch TV and Bea blocked my door and wouldn't let me in." I wasn't used to hearing Heather crying this way. "And also, Mama, Lori stepped on my eye as I was leaving school and my eye hurts too. I just wanted to go to my room. Mama, I don't want to stay with her."

Heather had never said that before. I felt suddenly helpless and pained, for Heather and for myself. I wanted to be able to go home and make it all better, put a Band-Aid on her soul, her day, her eye. In panic I told her she could come and stay with me in the hospital Thursday night.

Bea was by now calmed down. We agreed to talk about it in the evening when I got home.

Back at the OR sinks, scrubbing for the next case with Dr. Warren, I felt separated from work in a way I hadn't ten minutes before. I couldn't tell him of the crisis. Child-care issues stayed at home. Even more, though—nothing in his experience would give him empathy with what I was experiencing.

I was relieved to be back in the OR, scrubbed and ready to work, but I couldn't rid myself of anxiety about Bea's call. Was it true? Is Heather unmanageable? Has all this working and all these baby-sitters hurt her? Am I a bad mother? Will she hate me for having worked when she gets older? Thoughts usually easily dispensed with were coming through; my protection against them was shattered. I needed it to be okay at home and with Heather, so I could feel okay about myself.

I watched Irv Warren scrubbing the woman about to have an abortion and about to have her tubes tied. I wondered what he knows of women's lives.

Because this woman is a private patient, Irv does the procedure. He has a system of dilating the cervix: he puts the smallest dilator into the woman's vagina; I hand him the next largest size with my left hand, and with my right hand I remove the dilator which is still in the cervix. As I become absorbed in the rhythm of what we are doing, the phone call fades.

Wednesday   *Day 157*

Bea was apologetic. "Even as I blocked the door and wouldn't let Heather into her room, I thought to myself, Why am I doing this? She looks perfectly healthy and fine." She said she couldn't stop herself from carrying on that way.

As we all sat around talking about the afternoon, Heather added, "What Bea doesn't understand is that when I get home from school in the afternoon I'm tired and I need to go to my room to watch TV." Heather's eye is red but not seriously hurt. Apparently she fell going out the door, and then another child tripped and stepped on her eye.

Bea was also upset about the "popsicles" Heather ate—seven of them—but each was two ounces of orange juice I had frozen in Tupperware containers. So Heather had about fourteen ounces of orange juice, which, if consumed as juice, would have brought praise.

Perhaps all will be well, and today was just a difficult beginning.

Later

This morning at Grand Rounds, the woman whose Caesarean turned into a hysterectomy was discussed. She is still in the hospital, with an infection she contracted after the surgery. A small woman to start, she has lost fifty pounds and remains in unstable condition. She ignores her baby in the nursery, creating concern as to what she will do at discharge, assuming she survives. I heard a rumor that when they went in, they discovered that she might not have needed the section anyway.

Thursday   *Day 158*

Bea was up this morning at five, saying she had been sick to her stomach all night, and now had a severe headache. She wanted to take something strong for it, but I told her I only had aspirin, since I won't give anything stronger to someone I don't know well and for whom I am not serving as a physician. As I was leaving I noticed it was pouring outside. I asked Bea if she could walk Heather around the corner to school rather than sending her out the back over the slippery hill. She agreed.

I drove to work congratulating myself: "It's so wonderful that I have this house near the school. Otherwise I'd have to be worrying about Heather's being able to get to school in this weather." When I called home at four, Bea said, "I kept Heather home because of the weather. I took the authority to make the decision myself." Although I said nothing to her, I was furious that she hadn't called, that she first had agreed to walk Heather and then had felt free to do what she wanted. I had been so sure I had worked out all the problems at home, and now I had lost control over my life and Heather's again. I needed someone who would listen. I needed relief, and instead

I was getting bad surprises. And I was trapped in the hospital, where I still had twenty-two hours to go before I left.

The ER called me at midnight to see a woman who was bleeding. I came down and met Barbara, a black woman in her mid-twenties who was worried but still had a sense of calm about her. I liked her instantly, and felt her trust.

After taking a brief history, I examined her and found that her cervix was still closed, so her pregnancy might continue.

"Am I having a miscarriage?" she asked.

"It's still too early to tell. You might, or it might just be first-trimester bleeding. As long as your cervix hasn't opened, and you aren't having severe cramping, you may be okay."

"Is there anything you can do?" she asked, leaving me to answer what is hardest to say: "No. At this stage, if it's a miscarriage, you'll know soon. You'll have cramps and the bleeding will get worse." I felt so helpless, wishing I could meet her expectations and mine of what a doctor can do.

Before she left we had an exchange over her socks, which were identical to mine, the ones I'd finally found to make my feet more comfortable.

Saturday   Day 160

I'm on for another twenty-four hours. My parents will be arriving this afternoon to relieve Bea for the rest of the weekend.

The problem with Bea is complicated by her having been chosen by Fran and Laurie, leaving me worried that they will be angry with me if she doesn't work out. The thought of the loss of their support makes it even more difficult to sort out what is happening at home.

Yesterday afternoon, able to leave work early, I went home to sleep, telling Bea that Heather could wake me to say hello when she got home. Heather came in at three, but I went back to sleep immediately. Then she returned to wake me again.

"Mommy, can I make a cake for Gramma Emmy?"

"Sure, Heather, there's a mix in the kitchen cabinet."

"I know, but Bea said I had to come up and ask you if we could use it."

Bea feels free to keep Heather home for the day without consulting me, but can't use a cake mix without waking me after I've been up for two days. She seems, however, to be getting along with Heather, so I shouldn't complain. I'm not about to fire her, anyway. I can't take another change now.

Last night, instead of going back to sleep after dinner, I packed Heather up and went to Catherine's for a feminist meeting. Forever torn between my need for sleep vs. my need for contact with the outside world, I live on the edge of exhaustion.

Sunday   *Day 161*

Jackie and I went through our old routine today. She said I'm not working hard enough and that having part-timers is a drag. I told her I'm working more than I'd committed myself to, and that she has two people doing two-thirds time, which came to more than one full-timer.

Last night Barbara, the woman I saw Thursday night, returned. Her cervix had now opened, so spontaneous abortion was inevitable. When I examined her in the ER, I could see and feel the sac beginning to come through the dilated cervix.

With a sense of competence and purpose, I took Barbara to the OR for a D&C, which would now be done to prevent the hemorrhage which often is part of a miscarriage. The attending didn't even scrub in, but stayed in the room for the procedure and then left.

I painted Barbara with scrub solution in a style that was careful, thorough and gentle. I removed what was left of the products of conception, then gently scraped the uterus, without the usual violence. It was good to care about a patient and to feel that I could actually do something to help her.

Madeline is the new resident who replaced Bill ten days ago. I had avoided meeting her at first, afraid her start would be more difficult if she seemed to have been "contaminated" by me. Shortly after Karen started in the residency several months ago, she had said, "We shouldn't be seen talking to each other," and went off alone to a meeting to which we were both going. She spoke with me a lot in private, since I taught her how to run the unit, but she didn't want to be seen with me, even though we were friends and spent hours talking about house-decorating and children.

I met Madeline this evening, and agreed to come up to L&D to talk with her. She had many questions about the program which she was anxious to ask another woman.

I got to bed about one, but at two was awakened by a call from a nurse on L&D asking me to come up and help. The woman I was to check was having her first baby and was almost fully dilated when she arrived. I stayed for a while, thinking I might even stay with her for the delivery, but once the woman was fully dilated, the nurse began screaming at her to push, push, push, creating an atmosphere of hysteria. Feeling birth had once again been destroyed, I left.

I don't believe there is a second stage of labor. Labor is continuous. The baby moves down the birth canal at various rates depending on where it is and what the forces are propelling it. I can't help Madeline be a resident, because I no longer believe in the second stage of labor, so I can't teach her how to treat the "abnormalities," as they are defined here. There is no second stage.

Monday   *Day 162*

I'm back on for another twenty-four hours.

I have wonderful fantasies. I am up on Labor and Delivery saying to everyone, "But I don't believe in the second stage of labor."

I imagine I am in Dr. Pierce's office, saying, "But I don't believe in the second stage of labor."

"But it's real!" he tells me, showing me a chart of what it looks like.

"Yes, I used to believe in it. That's why I came here to study with you, but I don't believe it anymore."

"But it's right here," he tells me again, his finger vigorously pointing to Hill's chart, named after the man famous for establishing the standard labor curve.

"But it's not the system I believe in."

I don't tell him it isn't real, only that I no longer believe in it. His view of labor is his religious belief, but it is no longer mine.

Tuesday   *Day 163*

Last night Bea called to complain that Heather wouldn't eat her supper. Bea's hobby is gourmet cooking, but the food she prepares isn't anything Heather is used to. It is clear that none of this is going to work out unless I can get some time home, which is what I'm now trying to do.

I spoke with Jackie about shifting my hours so I can be home in the morning for a few days to work things out between Heather and Bea. Jackie expressed her disappointment in me, both in the hours I worked and in my "uninvolvement," as she described it.

I told her again about my dismay with what goes on in obstetrics.

"I don't think we do unnecessary Caesareans, though," she protested.

"That depends on what you call necessary, Jackie. I repeated what I've said before about the choosing of the baby's life over that of the mother.

"That's very heavy to think about," she said, looking thoughtful. "I'm scared to practice, Michelle. I feel locked into a certain kind of practice because I've never experienced it another way. You at least have seen other ways."

I sensed the absence of the usual barriers between us. Someone listening might even think we were friends.

"Jackie, I worry that in five years your practice will look like everyone else's, the only difference being that you are a woman." In the context of how it felt between us then, I didn't expect her to be threatened by what I was saying.

She went on to tell me how worried she was. "You know, four years ago when I came here, I thought the attendings were terrible, that what they did was terrible, but now I don't think they are so bad. I get along with them real well." Her statement had a question to it, but not one I could answer.

Nor could I answer for myself what I am doing here, subjecting myself at such personal cost to a system I see as bringing poor care to the patient and dehumanization to the physician. Part of me worries that in five years I will be saying the same words as Jackie.

Wednesday   *Day 164*

Being home for twenty-four hours has given me a chance to work things out with Bea. It was probably unrealistic to believe it could all go smoothly from the beginning when I was never home.

Heather is being difficult, cries easily and watches too much TV. I've put her on notice I will restrict it unless she cuts down on her own. I made up a new piece of cardboard with the phone numbers of Heather's friends, telling Bea that Heather needs help calling friends and arranging to play after school. This morning we decided on dinner—scrambled eggs and cooked carrots was what Heather wanted. We may do this on a daily basis.

Thursday   *Day 165*

Catherine called last night to say she wasn't feeling well. Heather was in bed and Bea was watching TV, so I decided to go over and take care of Catherine. I stopped at the supermarket, where I ran into Fran, who decided to join me. The three of us sat around talking and then we massaged Catherine to sleep, turned out the lights and left. The community of women here is exciting in the nurturing and being nurtured we offer and receive.

I keep thinking it will be better with Bea because she is nice to

Heather and seems to be trying, but this morning she told me she would be downtown all day. I reminded her that today Heather gets out of school at one. She said, "Oh yes," but I was left wondering what would have happened if I hadn't reminded her.

Also, all week I've been telling her that the garbage cannot be left in the yard because animals get into it. This morning I found the garbage strewn all over the yard. Bea said she would clean it up as soon as she got dressed, but then she left for the day without picking it up and I had to.

Later

The women who were to have prostaglandin abortions had come in, and since no one else was there to see them, I checked with the third-year resident and then began the insertion of the suppositories which would cause them to abort in the next twenty-four hours. When time isn't short I get genuine pleasure from my work; I can become fully engaged in taking care of someone. Even the trouble at home fades.

I did a D&C and laparoscopy this afternoon, the D&C showing a closed cervix, which is probably why the woman was having her problems. The laparoscopy showed nothing, which is what I had expected. Today's D&C was indicated, but I question the D&C for irregular bleeding. I can't understand how a hormonal disorder can respond to surgical intervention.

Putting someone in the hospital to have a D&C does seem to stop the irregular bleeding, at least for a while, but I'm not sure it's the D&C that helps. Of course, when cancer is suspected, doing a D&C gives you the opportunity to examine tissue. So often, though, procedures seem to be done "routinely" and thoughtlessly. This is not an atmosphere which encourages people to ask, "Are we doing the right thing?" or "Was this procedure necessary?"

I miss Carol because besides being friendly, she had the same perspective as I on how women should be treated. She's at another hospital, meaning that now there is no one here for me to talk to.

Chapter Eleven

Strict standards for doctors help to maintain good care, but they also exclude those people who challenge the system. In any hospital where I would practice, I would have to do Caesareans according to the standards of the hospital and the community at large. But what if those standards are wrong? What if the D&C is ridiculous? Unnecessary? Harmful?

I'm on duty now for another twenty-four hours. Heather is staying with Catherine until late this afternoon when Bea gets back, but I am apprehensive about any time they spend to-gether. Friday afternoon there was more difficulty, as Bea cooked food I asked her specifically not to cook, but forgot to put up Heather's hair, which she had promised Heather she would do before she left for the weekend.

I tried to tell Fran that it wasn't going well, but she didn't seem to hear me. I worry constantly about Fran and Laurie blaming me that things are not going well with Bea.

A woman who had a hysterectomy last week was complaining yesterday of vaginal pain. She had apparently not been told that her bladder had been punctured during the surgery, so she didn't understand why she was having urinary problems. She also didn't know that in order to remove the uterus and cervix, the vagina must be cut into. She and I had a long talk about the importance of women knowing what is being done to them. I will probably be chastised for talking so frankly to her.

My pager went off at eleven last night as I was hunting for x-rays on the pre-op patients. The ER nurse told me, "It's a bleeder, but I frankly don't see any blood." With obvious irritation at the patient, she added, "I don't think you have to rush down here."

After finishing my search for x-rays, I go down to the ER, and taking the chart from the rack, walk into the GYN room. A woman in her mid-forties sits on the table looking despondent, embarrassed and anxious.

"What brings you here?" I ask routinely, without paying much attention.

"I've been bleeding for a week, and it doesn't stop. I worry about something being wrong."

"How many pads do you use each day?" This is a good way to assess the severity of the bleeding.

"Two or three pads a day, I think, sometimes less." She looks down and away from me. "I mean, I know it isn't a lot of bleeding, but I'm worried."

I wonder if I will discover why she is here tonight. I'm only half listening as I jot down her answers to my questions: "When was your last period?" ... "How often do you get it?" ... "How long does it usually last?" ... "Are you sexually active?" ... "Do you use birth control?"

She answers them all easily but flatly. Then I ask, "Have you ever been pregnant?" She pauses and then I see that her eyes have filled with tears, her face is flushed and she begins to weep. Putting my paper on the chair where I've been sitting, I walk over to the table and stand next to her. There isn't much I can do except stand there, let her cry, and wait. For a minute I regret my previous distance and remoteness. I had been saving myself for the next ten patients, for the limitless demands on me here. I rest my hand on her shoulder to let her know I am there and that I can wait. Time seems to stop.

"I had a baby," she tells me between sobs as she looks around for a tissue, which I hand her. "I was fourteen and my family made me give it up and then I had another baby when I was fifteen and I gave that one up too. Every time I think of them I cry. I can't forget."

Handing her more tissue, I say, "Some pains don't go away, do they?"

"I keep trying to forget, but I never do. My babies are grown now, and I still can't forget them."

We then talked at length about adoption, what it is for mothers, for children. I told her about the adoption registry, about which I had recently learned, where women who have given up their children can register their names in case the children want to search for them. I said I would get more information about it for her.

As for her bleeding, I could find nothing on examination. I would guess it's of indeterminate cause and should just be watched for a while. Maybe it's bleeding from loss. Maybe it's the cry of her empty uterus.

Tuesday   Day 170

Last night Heather cried at bedtime and asked why I don't quit and why I have to work at night. She wants to move back to New Jersey, where I was so much more accessible to her.

I'm on my way in to work for another twenty-four hours, after having seen Heather off to school this morning. I stopped on the way to pick up a tape recorder for her, since recently she has been enjoying a recording I made of a children's story I once wrote. I want to record more stories for her to listen to at bedtime.

I feel terrible entering the institution, facing the silence of my life inside there, my isolation from the others.

Yesterday I spent five hours in the operating room reattaching tubes that had previously been cut. The attending let me do much of the case, using special operating eyeglasses which magnify the field. The patient was a woman who had her tubes tied several years ago, partly due to pressure from her doctor. She is having surgery done because she has remarried but also because she has always regretted the sterilization. There is a 30 to 50 percent chance of success, with an additional risk of future ectopic pregnancies. Most women are not informed of these facts before they have their "tubes tied." Before the surgery she and I spoke of sterilization abuses, and I told her I was in Washington last year to testify at HEW on sterilization abuses.

Thursday *Day 172*

I called in sick today, which is the first time off I've had in weeks, not preceded by a night in the hospital. I feel disoriented, unsure of the day of the week. My body hurts from the work I've been doing and the nights without sleep.

Saturday *Day 174*

Apparently past my initiation with the attendings, I was allowed to do a mini-lap, a laparoscopy, an open laparoscopy and an abortion yesterday.

Early in the evening I was asked to go in to see a woman who had a radioactive implant in her vagina. Since I was not convinced it was safe to go into the room, the nurse called down to radiology to ask for a lead shield. The radiologist said, "The shield won't do any good. Tell her to move quickly." The nurses have been told it is safe for them to spend half an hour per day in there. At rounds in the morning, I was told by Jackie and Richard that doctors are only to be in there for five minutes per day.

It is difficult to say "I am afraid." It is part of our training to deny dangers to ourselves. I knew a radiologist who boasted of never wearing shielding gloves for x-ray procedures. He died at forty-six of cancer.

Heather came in and stayed with me in the on-call room last night, so she is feeling better about my being in the hospital. I took her for a late snack in the cafeteria, and then to the OB floor so she could see where she might be able to stay with me sometimes when I go back on night OB. I was apprehensive about her being on OB because she has such a different view of childbirth from attending home births with me. I didn't want her to see the babies in the nurseries, or hear the women screaming, or even being yelled at. Once last year when she heard about a friend who was going into the hospital to have a baby she asked, "But what's wrong with her? Why does she have to go to a hospital?"

She slept in the morning while I made rounds, waking in time for us to leave.

Tomorrow morning I go on for thirty-six hours and work each day until Thursday, when I go back East to speak at a medical school on "Obstetrics and Gynecology: A Feminist Perspective." It will be a hectic three days back in New Jersey, my first visit since we moved.

This is also the end of the reduced schedule I was granted— late mornings to work things out at home. The crisis with Bea seems to have abated, but now I face the endless days of five o'clock awakenings.

Sunday   *Day 175*

The radiation technician here today refused to do the x-ray on the woman with a radioactive implant because she didn't want to expose herself to the risk. She went on to tell me, "You can't get a chest x-ray on her. By the time the film is carried through the room and put in back of the patient it will have been exposed. The radiation goes through everything."

We talked about technology in general, and she leaned over

and in a half whisper told me, "I had a roommate who had a baby at home and the baby was absolutely fine." I "confessed" to having attended home births.

Ultrasound uses radar-type waves to make a picture of organs and cavities within the body. It is currently being widely used on pregnant women to determine the location of the placenta and the size of the baby. It has never been proven safe. Articles have been coming out now for several years about possible hazards, but physicians have ignored the risk and presented this new method as "absolutely safe." It's frightening, because x-rays and DES were also thought to be safe. I talked with the technician about my concerns about ultrasound. She said, "All the radiologists know it does something. Male fetuses all get erections when exposed to the waves." I have read studies showing chromosome damage to cell cultures exposed to ultrasound. And the external fetal monitor, which we use so routinely, also employs ultrasound waves to record the heartbeat.

Ultrasound waves are also used to locate the placenta in order to perform amniocentesis. This is a procedure in which a needle is inserted through a pregnant woman's abdomen and into her uterus. Amniotic fluid, that which surrounds the fetus, is removed. Cells in the fluid are then analyzed for chromosomal abnormalities, as in Down's syndrome and other genetic diseases. This procedure is commonly performed on women over thirty-five years and when there is a familial history of genetic disorders. Both ultrasound and amniocentesis pose possible risks to the fetus.

My call home at six brought the discovery of new hassles with Bea, who insists that Heather is out of control. Bea doesn't want Heather to answer the phone or the door, both of which she has been doing for two years. I said I'd call and talk with her more after eight when Heather was asleep.

Then Heather got on the phone and talked with me about work again, asking me why I am working late at night.

"Someday, Heather, you may have to do something that isn't pleasant just so you can learn."

"I want to be a vet when I grow up," she told me.

"That sounds like fun."

"I want to help animals."

"You know, if you become a vet, you may have to work at night sometimes."

"I don't mind," she told me, "just so I don't have to be alone."

When I called home again after eight, Bea said they had also fought about closing the drapes of the living room. Heather had a friend over playing, and the girls wanted to close the drapes as part of their game. Heather insisted, then Bea exploded. Bea says, "If I can't determine when the drapes get pulled, then I'm not a person." I understand that Bea needs to feel that she and her work are important. Taking care of children in our society is considered such demeaning work that maintaining self-esteem can be difficult.

Even so, this long series of on-call nights, of which tonight is the last, has confirmed that I wasn't foolish in insisting on doing the program part-time. I've decided to leave Heather with my parents for her school-vacation week, since I don't want her home alone with Bea for a week.

It's midnight, and I'm standing in the on-call room looking out at the city and the empty hospital parking lot below. I haven't found a way to make my time here good for me. I have so many questions about the value of what I'm doing. The others in the program don't seem as troubled as I am, and this makes me feel distant from them and leaves me wondering about the years of training still ahead.

Tuesday   *Day 177*

Nanette, an eighteen-year-old, was admitted yesterday to be worked up for laparoscopy today. She has a long history of menstrual cramps and abdominal pain, and went through a laparoscopy before which showed nothing. When I expressed my doubts about another laparoscopy to her attending, he said he had to "do something" because she was calling him constantly. Today, before the surgery, when I raised the possibility of her problem being partly psychosomatic, he said, "But she seems like an honest person. I don't think she's making it up." I couldn't believe he thought psychosomatic means pretending. Psychosomatic pain is real, but it is the pain of the soul taken on by the body.

Today Nanette had needless surgery which showed nothing, while no one attended to the pain in her soul.

Dr. Brucker is a breast surgeon with whom I've been chatting in the OR lounge. He uses a technique of removing benign breast lumps under local anesthesia which he has offered to show me. Today I was able to get out of the laparoscopy in time to join him, so I have picked up one more skill.

Wednesday   *Day 178*

Lois Scott came up to me after Grand Rounds this morning and angrily asked, "Did you listen to Karen Reese's lungs this morning?" She is the woman whose ovarian cyst Lois and I removed a couple of days ago. This morning on rounds I saw that she had run a slight temperature yesterday, although by this morning it was normal. I found no site of infection.

"No, I examined her carefully," I told Lois, "but I guess I forgot to listen to her lungs."

Lois was outraged that I hadn't listened to the lungs of a patient two days post-op. I realized I hadn't listened because I knew they were fine. I asked Lois, "Did you hear anything when you listened?"

"No," she said, as I had expected she would.

I can't explain how I know, but sometimes I can just look at someone and tell if they are sick and where they are sick. I don't think I've ever missed a patient with a post-op lung problem. Usually I have a sense of where infection is, if it is present, and then the exam is to confirm what I already sense.

I agree with Lois, though, that I should have listened. That's what I'm supposed to be doing here and in any case, I should be monitoring my own instincts by taking all precautions.

One of my work-ups this afternoon was on a woman patient of Dr. Ingle's scheduled for a hysterectomy and removal of her ovaries in the morning. I went into her room, introduced myself, and said I would be asking her some questions and then examining her.

"What kind of examination are you talking about?" She seemed tense and apprehensive.

"I'll be doing a pelvic exam."

"No. I won't let you do that. I'll only let Dr. Ingle examine me," she protested defensively. She showed surprise when I said, "That's okay. I still need to ask you some questions."

I settled into a comfortable chair and she sat on the side of her bed while we talked. She was in her late forties, poised, well-dressed and quite open. She told me she had been having irregular bleeding, so Dr. Ingle said she had no alternative but to have her uterus removed. I thought there was a slight question in her statement but I wasn't sure. "I would wear a pad for the rest of my life if I knew I weren't in danger. It's not the bleeding that bothers me but the worry." The big fear for every woman is cancer, although this woman has the kind of irregular bleeding that often comes with menopause.

"Are your ovaries going to be removed too?" I asked, knowing already they were scheduled for removal, but wanting to check on whether she knew or had been included in the decision.

"Yes," she answered, looking at me again with some doubt in her expression. "Is there some question as to whether they should be?" We were discussing some of the pros and cons of ovary removal, of estrogen replacement, and the possibility of ovarian cancer if the ovaries are left in, when Dr. Ingle walked into the room.

"Oh, we were just sitting here talking about her ovaries," I said, looking up at him, hoping there was a chance this issue could really be discussed.

"That's not a question," he said to me sternly. "She decided that in the office and they're being removed, so that's the end of that." He turned to her, adding, "You know you won't let me

use hormones on you, so you have no choice about the hysterectomy." His manner was so imposing that this questionable con-
clusion took on authority.

Dr. Ingle read the "informed consent" statement, which lists
all the things that could go wrong, but I had the sense he was
only reading it because I was there in the room. For instance,
he said, " 'You understand there is the risk of perforation infection or bowel or bladder problems . . .' " The patient stopped
him, asking, "What, me? From this operation?" sounding
shocked. He then reassured her, saying he just had to read this
list, but for her not to worry about any of it.

"How uncomfortable will I be?" she asked, to which he replied, "Oh, not very bad. It's just a little operation."

"Will I be in agony?"

"Of course not. You'll have a day or two when it will hurt and
after that you'll be bouncing around and we'll have you out of
here in five days."

"Will I be able to do everything?" she asked, and I jokingly
responded, "You won't be able to ski the first week."

More seriously, Dr. Ingle told her, "You'll really be able to get
around in a week or two. You can drive, for instance."

It was all lies. She *would* be in agony after her surgery and
it would be weeks, even months, before she had her strength
back. And no one was telling her about the common changes
in sexual functioning after hysterectomy, the decrease in vaginal lubrication, difficulty in reaching orgasm, difficulty with
arousal.

Dr. Ingle explained to her that I would be doing a pelvic
exam on her. She said, "No. I'll only allow you to examine me."

"You have to let Dr. Harrison examine you," he told her, and
when it was clear she was going to refuse, Dr. Ingle looked at
me apologetically.

After he left, she was apologetic about her refusal. "There's
nothing personal about it. I just don't want anyone except my
doctor to examine me."

"It's not a problem for me. I respect and appreciate a

woman's refusal to have done to her what she doesn't want."

Her eyes were moist and so were mine. I felt moved by her need to defend the integrity of her body, and by her being apologetic about it.

With Dr. Ingle out of the room, she asked me, "What's the pain really like?"

"Most women have a lot of pain, but we write orders for a lot of medication the first few days, but you must ask for it."

"You mean they don't just bring it?"

"No, you have to ask."

"Then I'd better not just lie here and wait for it," she said, seemingly relieved by this useful information.

"We usually prescribe that it be given every three or four hours as long as you ask for it." I didn't want to scare her about the pain, but if she doesn't expect it, she will think it is because something has gone wrong, not understanding that this is a painful procedure.

She also returned to the question of having the hysterectomy. "Tell me, does the bleeding ever just stop?"

"Sometimes it does, but there is no way of being sure it will." I didn't know what to say because I sensed she had no real choice by then, and she needed to go ahead with her doubts settled. I was also afraid of Dr. Ingle. If the attendings perceived me as someone who interfered with their patients and challenged what they were doing, I would never be able to learn surgery. I thought this hysterectomy was ill-advised. I could see that the woman was still uncertain. But I felt I could say no more than I had already.

Her sister, who had left the room when I first introduced myself, returned. The patient said something about not being sure she wanted to go through with the hysterectomy, whereupon her sister said, "Well, I had a hysterectomy. Aren't I still the same? Don't I look normal?"

It was clear that no one would let this woman consider alternatives to this operation.

The days are getting longer again, so there are beautiful pale streaks in the sky and wonderful colors of daylight against the city skyline as I drive to work in the morning.

Barbara came to me in the locker room as I was getting into pinks, saying she wanted to do the hysterectomy I was scheduled to do with Doug Weston.

"Sure, Barb. It's okay with me," I said, much to her astonishment.

"You mean you'd do that for me?" she asked incredulously.

"Mostly I only displease people around here. Here's my chance to do something for you. I'll even cover the clinic for you if the case runs past noon." I remembered seeing Barbara holding the woman's hand in the pre-surgical waiting area, thinking to myself at that time that she should be the one doing the surgery, since she had done the work-up yesterday and was obviously close to the patient.

Jackie initially said yes to the switch, but then came to the OR to tell Barbara she couldn't scrub, and then sent for me. It seems that others had objected to someone of Barbara's first-year rank getting the case. In addition, Richard told Jackie he didn't want to have to work with me in the clinic, as he would if the case ran late.

I started the case with Dr. Weston, who ran into difficulty so that we soon needed another set of hands. Ironically, Barbara was called in to be second assistant, but once she scrubbed in, I moved over and let her be first assistant, which is what she had wanted in the first place.

By afternoon there was rampant anger among the residents. Jackie came to me at four looking tired and despondent, and said, "I suppose *you* hate me too."

"No, I'm not angry with you. I'm sorry everyone else is upset, but I'm not in it." I felt calm and relaxed as I spoke, able to be supportive of her. Being chief resident is a thankless task. Sometimes I think Jackie's cold and strident manner is all a protection against her natural desire to be liked by everyone.

Lloyd Stevens is an infertility specialist who has invited me to spend half a day a week in his office this spring. I'm very excited about doing that, although I certainly don't need extra work. I'll be on night OB then, and I'd go to his office one morning when I got off work.

It's six o'clock when I drive home. Although the sun has gone down, some streaks of light remain in the sky. They complete the day for me when I remember the beautiful pre-sunrise lightening of the sky as I drove to work.

Sunday   Day 182

Last Friday, speaking at the medical school in New Jersey, talking partly about my residency, I was struck by the youth and innocence of the students. Many came up to me afterward and asked, "How can we keep from becoming hardened?" They see students one year ahead already turning off, closing themselves, becoming dehumanized, so they are afraid. I have few answers for them other than that keeping contact with people outside medicine is important in maintaining values and perspective.

Tuesday   Day 184

Today I watched Doug Weston do a dilation and evacuation— the removal of a large fetus from the uterus. Richard had said the woman was thirteen weeks pregnant, but after she was under anesthesia Doug found an eighteen-week fetus. The procedure, under such circumstances, is gruesome, and extremely difficult for us as physicians. It is, however, much easier on the woman, who otherwise would have a saline abortion within twenty-four hours of labor before she passed the fetus. This way, she wakes up and it is over.

Doug Weston refuses to give pain medication to abortion patients, as does Jackie. Both of them insist that the pain is not as great as patients say. Weston also refuses to give pain meds to laparoscopy patients, who have a lot of pain after the procedure. We argued about medication over the sinks this morning as he tried to justify his practice. Although in OB I'm the one who questions medication, I see no reason not to give drugs for surgical pain.

"Pain medication should not be given, because of the possibility of masking a complication," he explained to me.

"I really disagree," I told him. "I don't think codeine would block the pain of anything serious."

"Michelle, I'm in charge. You have to do what I tell you," he said, pulling in his chin and stiffening his back as he spoke.

"I'm not disputing that, and I certainly won't write an order for pain meds when you don't want them, but I still disagree with your not using it."

Deepening his voice, he said, "I have great experience with such things, Dr. Harrison. You should not disagree with me."

"But I've practiced many years too, and I think the use of pain medication comes under the heading of style of practice, not of what is right and wrong."

Most of the morning he was in his usual bad mood, but while I was scrubbing a woman and prepping her for the abortion, I heard strange cooing sounds in back of me. Turning around I found the nurse rubbing Weston's neck and back.

"Was this a part of your job description?" I asked her, ostensibly as a joke.

She laughed and went on rubbing. I went back to draping the patient, and then, turning around to them, added, "I think this comes under the heading of sexual harassment on the job."

My remarks, although meant seriously, were understandably taken lightly, for it is expected that nurses will do what they can to improve the disposition of surgeons, who often behave erratically in the OR and who take out their bad mood on the nurses.

Dr. Weston was now feeling better, but apparently annoyed with me. He began boasting about his youth and being younger than me, half singing a song about thirty-five being "over the hill." I looked at Gert, one of the nurses who is thirty-six or thirty-seven, about my age, and I said to her in what was to appear light-hearted, "He's such a baby, what does he know at his age?," creating a sense of understanding and sisterhood between us.

Doug Weston retaliated with a diatribe against ERA. "I sure don't believe in it," he said. "I sure won't vote for it in this state."

Gert and I have talked a lot about child-care problems when we've run into each other in the dressing room. She had overheard my telling Jackie about my problems one day, and offered support. She and her children live nearby, and she has offered her two teen-agers as baby-sitters. Gert is divorced with five children. When they were younger and she had to be at work for the early-morning shift, she would wake one child at five and have that child stay awake in case of fire, or any other emergency, because she had to leave for work. She would rotate who had to be up each morning. She said she thought in some ways it was easier with five, because they had each other for company. It may be easier to leave five together, but meeting the needs of five children must be far more complicated and difficult.

Wednesday   *Day 185*

Joan, who will be starting as chief in a week, sat down and discussed the schedule with me. A mother herself, she seemed sympathetic to the problems I am having. I like her a lot. Her lack of anger is a relief here, but I wonder what she'll be like after three months of being chief.

Joan spoke at Grand Rounds about her months working in West Virginia, where she was the only obstetrician in the area. She had packed up her kids and her housekeeper and had gone off to experience rural medicine. After her talk and slide presentation she sat down next to me. Thinking how nice that was, I looked around to see if there were other seats where she could have sat. I began thinking how nice it was that someone would sit next to me even if there were other seats, suddenly tearful and aware of how alone and isolated I feel here. I wondered how the next three months would be, whether Joan would still be sitting next to me after that time, or whether my radicalness, my parttimeness, my general differences would bother her too much.

Maybe Joan and I can be friends now because we haven't yet worked together. In a different context I might be friends with many people here. In this setting, though, confronted daily by the institutionalized—though at times well-intentioned—abuse of women's bodies, it is impossible for me to "forget it" and be friends.

A psychiatrist friend of mine also spoke at Grand Rounds. During the discussion period I asked about possible long-term effects of ultrasound, which brought laughs from some of the attendings. Even so, it gave her a chance to talk about the issue, which is what I hoped would happen. I hoped they would listen to an "authority"—as they would not to me.

Thursday   Day 186

Between cases in the OR this morning I went to my locker and read a few pages from *Woman and Nature* in which Susan Griffin challenges what our society does to women. I hear her voice describing the operating room with organs being removed and women's bodies being "conquered" and disease being fought. Since I usually feel as if I am on a battlefield, her voice validates my imagery. I hear different voices from those around me; in her book I hear my voice valued.

I was late for sign-out this morning because I spent too much time taking care of patients on rounds. All Jackie can do is scream at me, and then scream louder. I'm weary of six months of trying and that it is still no easier, no more manageable. Yet it is the loneliness, the isolation that is worst.

Saturday   Day 188

Bea has had a week of paid vacation, since I had just hired her and hadn't known Heather would be away this week. Not wanting her in the house with me for the week, I decided to pay her, anyway. She called me yesterday at the hospital asking if there was anything she could do in the house before she returns

Sunday to take care of Heather. I told her she could come over and do some light housecleaning if she wanted to. Then I added, "I'll tell you what I would like you to do. I'm on for the night, so I'd love to come home to a bed made up with fresh sheets." As I spoke I could feel how inviting that bed would be after a night in the hospital. I saw myself getting into it in the morning, knowing Heather wasn't due back for another day, sleeping as long as I wanted. Bea said "Fine."

The night was very busy. I got only one hour of sleep and arrived home eager to go right to bed. I went upstairs to my room and there saw a bare mattress. The bed had been stripped but not remade. I broke down and wept. I would have been fine with the old sheets, an unmade bed, anything but a stripped bed left for me by the person who had asked how she could help. So I cried. Then I got angry. I made the bed but I couldn't sleep.

Bea came back to the house later in the morning saying she wasn't "into housework." She said I had spoiled the job because I wouldn't let her cook enough. She has given me thirty days' notice, although at the moment she isn't even talking to me.

Monday   *Day 190*

Heather arrived at the airport yesterday happy and eager to be home. She cuddled up to me in my arms, suddenly filling for me what had been missing all week. Heather's reaction to Bea's leaving was: "Now we'll have a fourth baby-sitter." I don't think Bea ever liked Heather, so for that reason it will be a relief to have her out of the house.

It is snowing lightly as I drive in for another thirty hours. The street lights have a glow because of the snowy air and the reflection of white on the ground. It is beautiful and quiet, with few cars. I always feel a closeness with other drivers at this hour, as though we are the lone partakers of the early morning.

I was to work four nights a week on OB, from eight at night to eight in the morning, but Joan and I figured out that I could work only two nights and still have the OB service covered, since the other two nights I was to work there would be overlap with Karen's time. I would then have the breather I need to spend some time at home. Not only do I have to work out child care, I have to work out first what I am doing in the program now and where I want to be in the future.

This evening Heather and I had a grown-up discussion about my being at the hospital so much in which she listed all the times I have been there in the past two weeks, saying, "It's not fair to me for you to work so much." I told Heather why I still didn't want to quit, but that I was trying to arrange my schedule so I'd be home more.

My talk with Joan left me feeling more optimistic about being able to stay. I have a meeting with Pierce tomorrow to discuss the change.

I told Dr. Pierce about the difficulties I was having.

"And do you have any solutions?" he asked.

"I know I don't want to quit," I told him, and he seemed both pleased and relieved. He said he had gotten some positive feedback both about my skills and my ability to get along with people. But, he added, without any warning, "I am putting you on a leave of absence."

"But, Dr. Pierce, I don't want a leave of absence," I protested. "Joan and I worked out a schedule that keeps the service covered and allows me to cut back to two days." I was fighting tears, not wanting to leave, not wanting this to be happening to me.

"I'm sorry, but you have no choice. It would be too destructive to morale to have you working less than the others." He was wrong. That may have been true in the past, but since Bea has been making so many calls to the hospital, the others have become fully aware of my child-care problems. If I work those two nights, no one would have to cover. If I leave, they will hate me more because someone else will have to do my work.

"Michelle, my only reservation about the leave is the loss of income to you."

He seemed surprised when I said, "It's actually costing me money to be here. I've been paying a hundred dollars a week plus room and board to baby-sitters. I take home five hundred dollars a month from the hospital and have to use my savings to allow me to stay here. If I don't work, I don't need a baby-sitter. It's not the money but the training I want."

Although I managed to hold myself together for the meeting, I spent most of the afternoon crying. Every time I spoke with anyone about leaving, I broke down. I kept going over what happened, trying to figure out how I could have done it differently, but I couldn't find any other solutions.

Joan said this evening at sign-out that she regretted my leaving because I had something unique and different to offer the program. Jackie, who was sitting with us, said, "It's a shame Michelle never had a chance to express her views."

Thursday morning   *Day 193*

There is no humanity in this system, not toward patients, not toward women who both work and care for their children. A part of me is still desperately trying to make it here, but, mostly I begin to realize I cannot mold myself into the kind of person who could. A battle rages within me between fighting to stay and seizing the offer of freedom.

Heather was thrilled when I said I'd be leaving work for a while. She ran to tell Bea, who then said to me, "If you're going to have kids, you shouldn't work at night. I know, because my mother did it." I suddenly felt pity for Bea, and thought about the many years she had harbored anger over the hours her mother had worked. In our society, child care consists of women pitted against other women in the struggle for time, money, recognition and gratification.

Friday morning   Day 194

It is possible that I cannot find a new child-care solution because I know I cannot stay in this program and I want relief from the daily battering to my sense of morality and integrity.

Medicine, particularly as it is practiced in the hospital, is a service industry that systematically and impersonally processes sick and healthy people. Physicians are trained and conditioned to see their patients as objects to be assembled and reassembled once they enter the system. If you are sick, or even if you are having a baby, you are presumed to be incapable of intelligent judgment, and therefore—quite properly—under the control of the experts.

The physicians, too, must fit the mold. Their ideas, their techniques, even their demeanor are processed by the system. It is by this same process that the system makes itself invulnerable —even to beneficial change.

Saturday   Day 195

I worked on night call with Joan. It was actually pleasurable because, for the first time since I worked with Carol, I wasn't alone. With the affinity I felt for her, it seemed simple: there was a certain amount of work to do, and we did it.

Yesterday morning, however, began with my doing abortions with Doug Weston, who was even more nasty and cutting than usual, but he has apparently been that way with everyone lately.

During one of the abortions he was sitting before the woman's vagina, inserting probes and mumbling half aloud, half to himself, that the residents here don't think they can learn anything from the attendings.

I reflected for a minute and then in a calm way decided to respond honestly. "I don't think that's the problem," I said. "I think you have a lot to teach, but sometimes you are so unpleasant that it's hard to learn anything from you."

He didn't seem offended by what I said, nor did he reply. Actually, he can teach us a lot. He is one of the developers of a new method of examining the inside of the uterus; other attendings come even from other hospitals to learn from him.

My latest fantasy is of taking off about six weeks, and somehow having child care in place by May so I can return—despite everything. On the other hand, when I can stop condemning myself for being a failure, I can enjoy the prospect of time in which to rest, think and write.

Sunday   *Day 196*

After Bea left yesterday—one week early—I spent the day exorcising her from the room she had used. First I cleaned the mess she left, and then I got some yellow paint from the basement and began painting. I hadn't expected to finish, but I did. I put up green gingham curtains I had brought from the New Jersey house and the room didn't seem the same anymore.

I was up on the ladder, feeling terrible about what was happening, wondering how I'd get through the week at the hospital that was still left, when I began to laugh. I suddenly looked at where I was, but instead of feeling the pain of separation and loss, I thought, What an interesting life you lead, Michelle!

Monday   *Day 197*

I made rounds Sunday morning, had about an hour of free time, worked nonstop until one this morning and then slept until five-thirty.

Last night I admitted a woman who came to the ER because of abdominal pain, weakness and fatigue for three weeks, but who is also severely depressed and was thinking of suicide yesterday. She hasn't slept in many nights, and may be hallucinating. I wanted to give her some sedation but my chief, Flo, who functions strictly by protocol, said we couldn't because the woman was admitted as a surgical case, so sedation was contraindicated. I didn't argue with her, but I knew what should have been done. With my impending departure, I find myself synthesizing what I know, and being able to be more certain about what I have learned and what I still need to learn.

I admitted a woman yesterday for hysterectomy who is a poor surgical risk. When I questioned her attending he said, "She can't use birth control because of her religion. I have no choice." I wondered whether she and her husband knew about the risks of the surgery she is about to have.

Wednesday   Day 199

Although I woke frequently during the night, I still feel rested this morning. Up at five, I sorted laundry, put away Heather's clothes, and cleaned up after Maggie, whom I forgot to let out last night.

Filled with sadness about leaving, I am also looking forward to time to write, time to myself. I fear I'll never go back because I'm not sure I could put myself through this again. I want to go swimming at the Y, to see my friends, to spend time with Heather. With spring and summer ahead, and some money left to live on, the possibilities seem infinite.

Afternoon

Tara, a neighbor, came to see me Monday because Brenda, her sixteen-year-old, was pregnant. They had been to an abortion clinic where they had been told that Brenda was actually nineteen weeks pregnant, not the eight she had thought. This meant she would have to have a saline abortion done in the hospital. I had hoped to do the procedure Friday morning because I would be on duty Friday night and could be with her when she aborted. I could also do a D&C to remove retained parts, if it was needed in the night. Since the soonest appointment for an admissions work-up was in two weeks—when I would be gone —I arranged to see Brenda today after I went off duty.

Tara and Brenda met me at noon in the clinic. It was officially closed at that hour, so we were free of time pressures. Brenda looked pregnant lying flat on the table with the pear-shaped bulge to her lower abdomen that is characteristic of a pregnancy of five months. I examined her both internally and externally, and although what I saw and felt seemed right for a pregnancy this size, something wasn't quite normal. I took a long time palpating, feeling, trying to imagine a baby inside there swimming around, but I couldn't "see" one in there. I didn't doubt that she was pregnant, but I couldn't find the baby. Although worried that I might upset either Brenda or Tara, I decided to listen for the heartbeat, which should have been present if the fetus was as large as Brenda's abdomen looked. I listened all over her abdomen, trying to hear a fetal heartbeat, trying to convince myself I heard one, but I couldn't hear it.

I told Tara something didn't feel right, so I wanted to establish fetal size by ultrasound examination. I was able to have the procedure done immediately. Watching as the technician made ultrasound pictures of Brenda's abdomen, we could see that she was only nine weeks pregnant. Two huge ovarian cysts had been mistaken for an advanced pregnancy.

I remembered that, some months ago, a woman was injected with saline for an abortion when she'd really had cysts—with almost fatal results.

In the evening

Depression has been with me all afternoon. Taking care of Brenda is what I want to be doing. I don't want to leave. While it's true that I look forward to all the other things I want to do, I want to be at the hospital. I'd like to be taking care of patients. But how I would like to be taking care of them better than this profession allows me to!

Thursday   Day 200

I went through the entire winter without ever being chilled, but for the past few days I can't seem to get warm no matter what I wear. It's warm out, but I'm chilled to the bone, in spite of a sweater, a shirt, my white jacket and a poncho. I didn't feel this way when it was six degrees out.

Friday   Day 201

Although yesterday I signed papers requesting the leave of absence, I still cannot believe I will be gone in the morning. A voice inside me wants to scream out in protest: "But you cannot take away my right to this learning, to these skills." They do not have the right to take away my work.

As I drive to the hospital for these final twenty-four hours, I keep looking for a different ending.

Saturday   Day 202

After sign-out, when everyone was leaving for the night except Flo and me, Charlie, who has always been so friendly, walked by and said, "Well, I guess I won't see you. Bye." He suddenly made real what I hadn't fully believed. My fantasies of being rescued were not happening.

Joan said, "I'm sorry it ended this way. Call me if it gets unbearable." I was in tears by now with all my reserve gone.

I kept trying to get myself together. Fortunately I wasn't being paged to go anywhere, so I could hide out in the on-call room. I sat on the bed grieving, not having the energy for one more night of battle in a war that had already been lost. I was to surrender in the morning, but I was ready to give up now. Overwhelmed by a sense of failure, I wanted to be able to slip off to lick my wounds in private. I wanted to go home.

For one of the few times since Heather's birth, I felt incredibly alone with her. I was her only parent, but she was also the person closest to me in the world. I wanted to be holding her.

At eleven I went to the ER, which by now had patients for me to see. As usual, being with a patient put distance between me and my own pain. Alone in the room, working with my hands and my mind, offering comfort, time seems to stop as I become totally immersed in what I am doing.

The first patient I saw was a young pregnant woman, terrified, crying, writhing with abdominal pain, probably as a result of the Chinese dinner she had just eaten. Speaking with her, and then examining her, I felt her begin to relax while the pain seemed to subside.

"I think your hands have healed her," the surgical resident was saying. "I've noticed you doing that before."

Sometimes I can feel my hands making someone better. I also at times "know" in my fingers what is wrong. Flo came down, and after seeing the woman, said, "Michelle, do whatever you think on her. I've learned not to disagree with you about abdominal pain," referring to a disagreement we'd had early this week about another woman.

By three o'clock in the morning, after seeing two more patients in the ER, and then stopping up on L&D, this time ready to say goodbye, I was able to return to the on-call room to sleep.

I dreamed I was sitting at the piano, trying to play, but just as my fingers began to move freely and the notes became music, a giant metronome would begin to tick at a slightly different rate. I kept trying and trying to play, but each time I felt the music begin to flow out of the piano, the metronome would change again, confusing me, stopping my fingers.

Awake at six, I made rounds, then signed out to the people coming on duty for the day.

Heather threw herself in my arms this morning when I went to pick her up at Catherine's, and then decided to stay and play with her children Alex and Chrissy for the day. I held her, though, for a long time, reassuring myself that she was all right, that she too had survived.

I spent the day grocery shopping, doing laundry, getting my house in order, wondering what I was going to do next, but still engrossed in what seemed like an unfinished dream. I thought of my visit to L&D last night, when I listened to the roar of the galloping fetal monitors, and I understood for the first time why the technology interferes with childbirth: birth is a creative process, not a surgical procedure.

I picture dancers on a stage. Once, doing a pirouette, a woman sustained a cervical fracture as a result of a fall; she is now paralyzed. We try to make the stage safer, to have the dancers better prepared. But can a dancer wear a collar around her neck, just in case she falls? The presence of the collar will inhibit her free motion. We cannot say to her, "This will be entirely natural except for the brace on your neck, just in case." It cannot be "as if" it is not there, because we know that creative movement and creative expression cannot exist with those constraints. The dancer cannot dance with the brace on. In the same way, the birthing woman cannot "dance" with a brace on. The straps around her abdomen, the wires coming from her vagina, change her birth.

The birthing woman plays in an orchestra of her body, her soul, her baby, her loved ones, her past and her future. And we do not know who leads the orchestra.

Doctors cannot lead the orchestra, because they are not within the process. Unable to hear the music, trained only in modalities of power and control, they can only interfere with the music being played.

What should they be able to do? They should stand ready to help the player in trouble to get back into the rhythm. Instead, they take over. Instead of supporting the mother, they say, "Okay, you have failed. It's our piece now."

How do you get a 30 percent Caesarean-section rate? You orchestrate it. You write a piece in which the third movement is a Caesarean, then build the first two with that in mind. You write in a different language; you write in terms of centimeters of dilation, external fetal monitor, internal fetal monitor, pH, scalp electrodes, Caesarean-birth experience, arrest of labor, protracted labor, fetal distress, episiotomy, prolapse, cephalo-pelvic disproportion, ultrasound waves, amniocentesis, "premium baby," post-mature (when the baby stays too long in utero) and "maternal environment" (formerly known as the mother). Those are the words, the notes, while the piece is played to the rhythm of fear.

Epilogue

I didn't go back. Fran, Laurie and Catherine were ready to help in child care again, while Heather was looking forward to another baby-sitter. Although it was the child-care problems that had precipitated my leaving when I did, I chose not to return to Doctors Hospital. Making that decision was a slow and difficult process.

Initially I was overwhelmed by a sense of defeat and by self-accusations of "not being able to take it." I thought, If only I had tried harder. I had let down the women who had supported me, the midwives who hoped to practice with me, and myself. I had overestimated my strength and underestimated my vulnerability.

In the months that followed my leaving, as I tried to explain what happened, I came to feel that I had been fighting a war which no one else even knew existed. I couldn't face going back to the loneliness of my life on the front line. My friends could only come with me as far as the door of the hospital or be at the other end of the phone—when I could call. I had wanted to be a more sensitive and skilled physician, not a soldier learning to be hard, to distance myself, to attack organs and intact tissues. I didn't want to be in pain. I also didn't want to be creating pain.

When I returned to training more than ten years after my first medical school rotation on OB-GYN, I thought I could more easily accept the compromises that were necessary, and indeed for a while that was true. But the same conflicts were with me. I couldn't say indefinitely, "Well, I'll just do these things for four years and then I won't have to . . ." I didn't trust myself, because one can always find "reasons" to justify immorality: there are standards, peers, economics. Once justified, they no longer seem so bad. I was afraid that the lures which had caught the others would snare me too—that I couldn't take just a little of the poison.

If we murder we are murderers. If I take out a uterus that need not be removed, if I cut a perineum that need not be cut, then I am committing those crimes. The tissue is no less cut, nor the organs less removed because I, as a woman, am wielding the knife. The poison of OB-GYN is no less lethal when dispensed by a woman.

If I were to have an eye removed, then I would forever be a person with only one eye. If I were to take in poison without spitting it out, I would be a poisoned person. I might survive, but I would be damaged. Medical training is no less violent than surgery or poisoning. It leaves women and men no less scarred or no less without the organs that have been removed.

Medical training works like brainwashing. Two major components are sleep deprivation and isolation from one's support system. Because I was part-time, I was not so cut off from my support nor so deprived of sleep as the other residents. Single-motherhood made it both less desirable and less possible for me to remain separate from my life outside the institution. In addition, my feminism gave me a political context in which to see what was happening to women in the hospital. A combination of both my personal circumstances and my political perspective made it easier for me to challenge what was being told to me, although it took the distance of leaving to be able to see clearly what I was doing and what was being done to me.

Closed off from feeling, I was at times cold as the green walls around me, cold as I had feared before I returned to hospital childbirth. People had become characters in my life. A woman baby-sitting in my home, suffering the pain of her own childhood, was treated by me only in terms of her function in my life. I needed her to take care of Heather, to ask no questions, to insulate me from her needs and those of my child's. Why? So I could take out uteruses and ovaries and wear the uniform of power and acceptance. All day I could perform heroic deeds and be thanked and respected as a humane physician, but in truth I did not function humanely. I was removed from my own gentler self by this ungentle profession.

Would I practice again? At first I thought I had said goodbye to medicine. I sold the house so I would have money to live on, uprooted myself and Heather, again moved back East and concentrated on the writing of this book. For the next two years I wrote, practiced some psychotherapy and studied areas now being called holistic health.

Gradually I have moved back into practice because I remain committed to it as well as to trying to integrate conventional medicine with my visions of how it ought to be.

Women need good health care. The future of women's health care, however, does not lie in the domain of current obstetrics and gynecology, which is founded on certain assumptions about women's bodies and women's lives. Contemporary medicine is based also on the belief that machines are as accurate as humans, that data can be hard, that numbers and statistics and graphs can faithfully represent a human being. This kind of practice excludes intuition, sensitivity and mutuality. It thereby deprives both the physician and the patient of their power to heal and be healed.

I used to have fantasies at Doctors Hospital about women in a state of revolution. I saw them getting up out of their beds and refusing the knife, refusing to be tied down, refusing to submit —whether they are in childbirth or when they were forty and having a hysterectomy for a uterus no longer considered useful. Women's health care will not improve until women reject the present system and begin instead to develop less destructive means of creating and maintaining a state of wellness. It is my hope that this book is a step in that process.

EXPLANATION OF MEDICAL TERMS
USED IN THIS BOOK

abortion Termination of a pregnancy prior to about twenty weeks gestation. It can be spontaneous (a miscarriage, in lay language) or induced—that is, the result of deliberate interference with the pregnancy.

Stages of abortion
1. Threatened abortion: vaginal bleeding present with little or no cramps, cervix is closed.
2. Inevitable abortion: vaginal bleeding, cramping, with some dilation of the cervix.
3. Incomplete abortion: part of the products of conception (fetus, membranes, placenta) have been expelled through the uterus, but part (usually the placenta) remains in the uterus.
4. Complete abortion: fetus, membranes and placenta have all been expelled.

Types of induced abortion
1. Suction abortion: the cervix is dilated and a suction hose used to remove fetal parts.
2. Saline abortion: saline (salt) solution is injected through the abdomen of the woman and into the uterus, resulting in labor and abortion within about twenty-four hours.
3. Prostaglandin abortion: suppository of prostaglandin, a hormone, is placed in the vagina to induce labor, and abortion then usually occurs within twenty-four to thirty-six hours.

abruptio placenta Premature detachment of the placenta from the uterus which can result in fetal death and maternal hemorrhage.

adhesions Thin bands of tissue like filmy spider webs attaching organs and structures to each other in the abdominal cavity.

amniocentesis   Insertion of a needle through the uterus and into the amniotic sac of the fetus to remove amniotic fluid for study.

anterior/posterior repair   Repair of the mucosa or wall of the vagina and surrounding tissue for purpose of resuspending bladder (in the case of cystocele) and correcting the loosening of tissue between rectum and vagina. The operation is often performed for purpose of tightening the vaginal opening.

bili-light   When a jaundiced newborn is exposed to either artificial or window light, there is a breakdown and excretion of the bilirubin which has caused the jaundice. The light used in hospitals is called a bili-light because it is used in the treatment of excess bilirubin.

breech   When fetal position is such that buttocks or feet are in position to be delivered first.

Bartholin cyst   Common disorder of Bartholin glands of vagina, often requiring draining and occasionally removal of the entire cyst.

cauterize   To burn tissue either with chemicals or electrical heat. Used when cervix is inflamed; used also in surgery to stop bleeding of small vessels instead of tying them with sutures.

cephalopelvic disproportion (CPD), or head-pelvis disproportion   When the fetal head size is estimated to be larger than the pelvic opening through which it must pass. It is usually measured by x-rays.

clinical cephalopelvic disproportion (clinical CPD)   When x-rays show there is room for the fetus to pass but because of failure of labor to progress, CPD is judged to be present on clinical grounds, i.e., by observation.

colposcopy   Use of portable examining microscope to look at the cells of the surface of the cervix and vagina. It is used to locate abnormal cells, especially in DES daughters.

curettage Scraping of the inside of a cavity. In GYN it is the scraping of the lining of the uterus. *See* D&C.

cystocele A bulging of the bladder into the vagina. May be mild without symptoms and found only on examination, or may produce urinary incontinence.

D&C Dilation, or widening of the cervix, and then curettage, or scraping of the uterus.

DES (diethylstilbesterol) An estrogen that was frequently given to pregnant women twenty to thirty years ago to prevent miscarriage. It has been found to cause cancer and other severe deformities in the reproductive tract of female offspring, as well as deformities in the reproductive tract of male offspring. DES was apparently never effective in preventing or stopping miscarriage. DES is also given to women as the "morning-after" pill.

ectopic pregnancy Pregnancy that occurs outside the uterus, most commonly in the Fallopian tubes. When it ruptures, there can be severe hemorrhage.

epidural anesthesia Anesthetic drug that is injected through a catheter, or tube, which has been inserted in the outer portion of the spinal canal. The tube allows continuous or repetitive doses of the medication, thus extending the duration of the anesthesia effect.

episiotomy Incision of the perineum of a woman in order to enlarge the vaginal opening during childbirth. Two main types are *median,* which extends downward toward the anus, and *mediolateral,* which extends downward but off to one side of the anal sphincter.

fibroids Benign growths in the walls of the uterus, a frequent cause of irregular bleeding. They can grow quite large or be small and without symptoms. They usually regress with menopause.

hydrosalpinx Collection of fluid in a Fallopian tube, often a result of previous infection.

hysterectomy Removal of uterus, done either vaginally, *vaginal hysterectomy,* or abdominally, *abdominal hysterectomy.* Removal of ovaries is *oophorectomy.* Removal of Fallopian tubes is *salpingectomy.* Removal of uterus, tubes and ovaries is *hysterectomy with bilateral* [both] *salpingo-oophorectomy.*

IUD (intrauterine device) Plastic or metal device placed inside the uterus to prevent conception. Frequent complications include perforation through uterus and into the abdomen, increased bleeding, pain and infection.

jaundice A yellow staining of the skin and organs resulting from build-up of bile in the system. It is common in newborns, and depending on the etiology of the jaundice, may or may not be serious.

laparoscopy Surgical procedure in which tubes and light source are inserted into abdomen for purpose of visualizing pelvic organs and for ligating of Fallopian tubes.

laparotomy Surgical incision into the abdominal cavity.

lithotomy Used in GYN to denote a woman's position on a table with her legs up in stirrups and spread apart, giving maximal exposure to her labia and perineum.

meconium The first fetal bowel movement, which is sometimes excreted in utero if the baby is stressed. The amniotic fluid then becomes stained, referred to as *meconium staining.*

mini-lap Modification of a laparotomy involving a very small incision in the abdomen. Used for tubal ligation during sterilization.

myomectomy Surgical removal of fibroids from the walls of the uterus.

pessary A device of rubber, plastic or metal placed in the vagina to push up a uterus that is sagging down.

Pitocin A powerful drug given to begin or stimulate uterine contractions when delivery of a fetus is desired. It is also given after a delivery to help uterus to contract and thus decrease bleeding.

placenta previa Placenta is implanted over the cervix either partly or completely, thus blocking the fetus from being born vaginally. A Caesarean section is then life-saving for both mother and fetus.

premium baby Term used to denote a baby of a woman over thirty-five years of age (considered elderly in OB) or the baby of a woman who has had previous infertility.

prolapsed cord The umbilical cord protrudes through the dilated cervix ahead of the baby so that baby's head descending into the birth canal presses the cord and prevents blood flow to the baby, with subsequent fetal death.

prolapsed uterus Uterus which has lost some of its muscular support and protrudes into the vagina, either moderately with few symptoms or in severe cases actually outside the vagina.

rectocele Protrusion of the rectum into a portion of the vagina. May be mild, without symptoms, or severe, with constipation and difficult defecating.

ruptured membranes When the amniotic membranes surrounding the fetus are broken, thus allowing the amniotic fluid to leak or spill out. Once the membranes are ruptured in labor, both fetus and mother are more susceptible to infection.

true knot When the umbilical cord becomes tied into a knot, which is then pulled tight as the baby descends through the birth canal, thus stopping the blood supply to the baby and resulting in death.

ultrasound The use of sound waves of high intensity to make a picture of internal organs, similar to sonar. No long-term studies have demonstrated its safety. Used in OB to locate placenta and estimate fetal size. It is also used in the external fetal monitor and hand-held amplifying fetal stethoscopes.